DR. PAUL A

CANCER

. . .

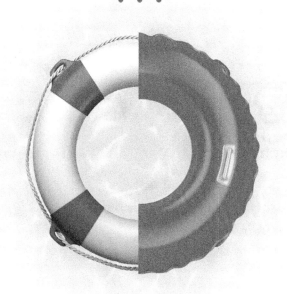

THE JOURNEY *from* DIAGNOSIS
to EMPOWERMENT

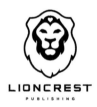

LIONCREST
PUBLISHING

CANCER

The Journey from Diagnosis to Empowerment

ISBN   978-1-5445-1600-4 *Hardcover*

      978-1-5445-1599-1 *Paperback*

      978-1-5445-1598-4 *Ebook*

There are two forces that allowed this book to come to be: my wife, Lori, for her enduring support and the thousands of patient stories and interactions that taught me the true depth of this work.

CONTENTS

FOREWORD

AN INTRODUCTION TO
CANCER: THE JOURNEY FROM
DIAGNOSIS TO EMPOWERMENT
BY BRUCE H. LIPTON, PHD

Quantum physics, the most valid of all of the sciences, recognizes that consciousness shapes our life experiences. In spite of its implications for human existence, this profound awareness has not become part of our everyday world. In contrast to consciousness controlling life, the public has been programmed with the belief that genes control the character of their biology, behavior, and emotions. With the belief that genes "turn on and off" in controlling their activity, we are left with the realization that we are "victims" of our DNA.

In the early 1990s, the science of heredity was completely revised with the introduction of *epigenetics*. This new science reveals that gene activity is controlled by the environment and, more importantly, by our *perception* of the environment. Epigenetics is the science of "mind over body." The perceptions and thoughts we hold in our mind are translated into complementary chemistry by the brain. Once released into the body, these neurochemicals control behavior and genetics. In light of epigenetics, both physics *and* biology now emphasize that consciousness shapes our reality.

Does the mind really control biology? The answer to that has been known for nearly a hundred years as revealed in the *placebo effect*. Most people are aware of this effect, wherein a placebo sugar pill induces healing. In reality, the pill did not engage healing; it was the patient's *belief* in the pill that healed them. The placebo effect illuminates the fact that positive thinking can heal almost any disease.

What about negative thinking? Most people do not realize negative thinking is equally powerful as positive thinking in controlling our lives; however, it works in the opposite direction. Negative thoughts engage the *nocebo effect*, a consciousness that can manifest any disease, even death. Stress, the primary consequence of nocebo's negative thinking, is responsible for up to 90 percent of disease, whereas defective genes are associated with only about 1 percent of disease.

The positive and negative thoughts controlling life experiences are derived from consciousness, a function attributed to the activities of the conscious and subconscious minds. The primary seat of the conscious mind is the prefrontal cortex, a lobe of brain tissue behind the forehead. The conscious mind is the *creative* mind associated with our source or spirituality. The subconscious mind represents a stored database of programmed instincts and acquired behaviors referred to as habits.

If consciousness is creating our life experiences, then why do our lives not match the wishes and desires we hold in our creative conscious mind? Science has revealed that only 5 percent of our life is controlled by the conscious mind, whereas 95 percent is under the control of programmed habits in the subconscious mind.

The primary programming of the subconscious mind occurs between the last trimester of pregnancy and age seven. During this period of development, the child's brain is predominantly operating at an EEG frequency referred to as *theta*, a state functionally expressed as hypnosis. As children, we learn basic human behavior by simply observing and downloading the behaviors of parents, siblings, and community. During this period of development, humans acquire their greatest fear— the fear of death.

In light of this awareness, consider the impact a cancer diagnosis has on the mind of a patient. It is one of the most primal of all stressors, for it confronts the patient with their greatest fear—death. In the minds of most patients, cancer diagnoses give rise to threatening end-of-life images including incapacitation, pain, and an ending. In conjunction with conventional beliefs regarding genetic control, cancer patients perceive themselves to be powerless victims of runaway genes.

In the patient's mind, a cancer diagnosis generates a nocebo effect that will manifest the deepest and darkest thoughts of their bleak prognosis. In contrast, consider the consequence if the same patient would invoke the placebo effect. Their mind would engage a positive healing influence that would offer a longer, happier life, and in some cases, even lead to a remission of the cancer.

How can cancer patients consciously take charge of their fate?

The answer is provided in *Cancer: The Journey from Diagnosis to Empowerment* by physician-scientist Dr. Paul S. Anderson. Supported by decades of experience as a cancer palliative provider, his book offers cancer patients a life-changing compilation of professional experiences that reveal how thoughts and emotions profoundly influence their prognosis.

Anderson's research emphasizes that the decision as to how to process a cancer diagnosis is completely up to the patient. Of all the factors that affect the prognosis, choosing to embrace the empowerment offered through mental and emotional work is perhaps the most significant. Anderson illustrates the power of his message by comparing the case files of two patients: Gia, who responded to her leukemia diagnosis with a placebo-engaging positive consciousness, and Bob, who responded to his pancreatic cancer diagnosis with a nocebo-negative consciousness.

Central to the mission of *Cancer: The Journey from Diagnosis to Empowerment* is Anderson's assessment that the prognosis of cancer patients and their support team is predicated on how they navigate through the five stages of grief as described by Elisabeth Kübler-Ross: denial, anger, bargaining, depression, and acceptance. Years of engaging with his cancer patients led Dr. Anderson to recognized that the manner in which patients consciously process their diagnosis profoundly influenced their outcomes, quality, and quantity of life. Patients who work through grief's emotional stages have profoundly more control over their prognosis than those who remain stuck in one or more of Kübler-Ross's stages.

On the upside, Paul Anderson's research offers readers a new and empowering sixth stage of healing grief—*hope*. Once a patient comes to terms with the current fifth stage of grief—acceptance—Anderson provides insights and protocols to enable the patient to transcend the diagnosis and take control of their health.

Cancer: The Journey from Diagnosis to Empowerment offers patients and caregivers an opportunity to move beyond misperceived limitations and write new, empowering stories for themselves and the world. Now, let the healing begin.

Bruce H. Lipton, PhD, is a stem cell biologist, epigenetic science pioneer, and best-selling author of *The Biology of Belief*, *Spontaneous Evolution* (with Steve Bhaerman), and *The Honeymoon Effect*. Bruce is a recipient of the prestigious Japanese Goi Peace Award in recognition of his outstanding contributions toward the realization of a peaceful and harmonious world for all life on Earth.

INTRODUCTION

You have, or someone you care about has, been diagnosed with cancer. Now what? The diagnosis could have been today or a year ago; ultimately, it doesn't matter. The process of living with one of the most feared diagnoses can be difficult, enraging, confusing, and many other feelings—but there is hope.

You, as the person with cancer or the person who cares about them, can be confused or angry because of the loss of control over almost everything you feel—an emotional soup that may be different every day. This confusion (or emotional soup) is aggravated by the fact that nobody wants a cancer diagnosis.

This is completely normal. The combination of emotional responses and confusion can lead to a mental drifting that can sabotage your health. The drifting starts from many thoughts, feelings, and emotions crashing in on you, and you cannot process, sort out, and move past it all. You feel lost because you have seen or heard about so many people with cancer, some who do very well and some who do horribly. You may feel stuck not knowing if anything you do really matters.

HOW CAN THIS BOOK HELP?

The goal of this book is to use the many years of experience I have had with patients and loved ones dealing with cancer and provide you with the tools you need to navigate this difficult terrain. Why? Because the better your internal journey (mental/emotional or mental/emotional/spiritual—whichever you prefer), the healthier you will be, the better your quality of life will be living with cancer, and the outcomes from any medical intervention will generally improve as well. Yes, the internal journey makes that much difference.

This all sounds good, but you might ask, "Why should I trust you and your advice?"

This is the most important question to ask first. My passion for the topic and drive to write this book comes from living this journey daily in my practice with people who have cancer and those who love them. My experience in medicine goes back to my work as a laboratory technician starting in the late 1970s. I later decided to finish medical school and went into practice as a family doctor practicing integrative medicine. Early in my practice, patients with cancer started to approach me, not for cancer therapy but rather for "quality of life" care. This included dealing with cancer or therapy-related side effects as well as helping them heal after surgery, chemotherapy, and other procedures. We also began to help people with diet, lifestyle, and other advice, as well as navigating the many natural therapies they were considering.

Later in my career, I was involved in a five-year cancer research project funded by the National Institutes of Health, which looked at whole practice integrative oncology and the potential to support patients and extend quality and length of life.

At the end of that research stint, a colleague, Dr. Mark Stengler, and I wrote a book called *Outside the Box Cancer Therapies* (Hay House Publishing). We are humbled daily as we still hear how that book is changing lives. *Outside the Box* eventually went on to become an international best seller, but I believed something was missing.

In *Outside the Box*, we focused on the therapeutic aspects of treating and supporting the patient with cancer. The book is a resource for what works and the reasons why they work in the integrative oncology world. It is an excellent resource for almost all of an individual's cancer journey. We had focused *Outside the Box* heavily on integrative therapies for cancer, how to use integrative oncology to heal from and improve the success of standard treatments, and other "physical" issues (e.g., what causes cancer, how do I prevent cancer, etc.), but we had only limited space in *Outside the Box* for the internal journey and the incredible impact it can have on health, survival, and other aspects of cancer.

Whether you prefer "mental/emotional" or "mental/emotional/spiritual" in reference to the internal journey, the book you are now reading is devoted completely to the internal journey and its bearing on your overall health and quality of life during cancer.

WHY ANOTHER BOOK?

In a review of the years of patient experiences, I saw three things that were critical to survival beyond the typical cancer therapies (e.g., chemotherapy, surgery, radiation therapy, and many integrative therapies). The three other factors that independently affected survival, quality of life, and thriving with cancer were what and how you eat, the care you provide your physical body, and the mental and emotional work you do. After seeing that our book *Outside the Box* did well at addressing the first two factors, it became clear that a book aimed at the mental and emotional process was necessary.

In the pages that follow, we will look at how this internal work can affect you and your health, areas to watch out for that can trip you up, and straightforward ways to make the journey positive. This book is for anyone who wants to improve their internal work around their own or a loved one's cancer diagnosis. It is written to be easy to read and implement. I have specifically kept the information short and to the point because, as you will see, there are some things you may already do quite well and many you may not be aware of. I want you to gain benefit from the book as quickly as possible without long "deep dives" into highly technical processes. There are countless resources for "deep dives" into any topic I bring up in the book; no need to repeat those (plus the book would be 1,000 pages if I did!).

So please use this book to become more aware of the process, more aware of tools and resources available, and to identify areas you want to learn more about and delve into more deeply. It is designed for you to quickly assess where you are and locate resources to get to the next step.

The way you mentally and emotionally process matters.

By now, I've spent more than twenty years practicing palliative oncology (helping people improve quality of life during and after cancer treatment) and integrative oncology (blending the best that modern Western medicine and other medical traditions and sciences have to improve outcomes for people with cancer). Throughout this time, I've seen countless patients, counseled numerous families and friends, and observed the impact the inner landscape of the mind can have. I have seen many people deal with cancer. I've facilitated better quality of life for my patients and helped them with life-extending therapies. I've coached them through some rough times. I've also walked with people through remission and through their end-of-life process.

There are no easy days when dealing with cancer. But time and again, I've seen that the way we process everything, from the life-altering diagnosis to therapy to uncertain outcomes, can literally make or break everything else.

So this book is my long experience interwoven with science and real-world outcomes with the goal to empower you to make the best of this journey.

A brief note about references:

Throughout the book, and in the Resources section at the end, I have books, websites, and other resources listed in standard reference format to make it easier for you to locate them. In the chapters, I do quote from a few peer-reviewed scientific papers. Rather than use the typical scientific reference for these quotes, I have referenced them with their PMID number. This is their identifier on PubMed, which is an online scientific reference library. If you are interested in any of those papers, type "PubMed" into your search bar, and the link will come up to the PubMed home page (https://www.ncbi.nlm.nih.gov/pubmed/). Type the PMID in the search bar, and you will be taken to the paper I quoted.

If you have read this far and are still interested, this is the book for you. Let's start the journey to discover how your mental and emotional state can dramatically impact your cancer journey and health!

CHAPTER 1

A CANCER DIAGNOSIS IS LIFE CHANGING

HOW WE DEAL WITH IT MAKES A DIFFERENCE

"We must be willing to let go of the life we've planned, so as to have the life that is waiting for us."

—JOSEPH CAMPBELL

THE STORY OF BOB AND GIA

GIA'S STORY

Gia woke one morning deciding she needed to act on the nagging feeling deep within her. For a number of months, she had not felt like herself and inside knew something was wrong. She seemed more and more tired, and the vitamins she was taking to help her energy didn't seem to be doing anything. She had turned fifty-seven two months ago and had enjoyed lifelong good health. Her family was healthy, except for one aunt who died of lung cancer after a life of heavy cigarette smoking. As for the rest of the family, not only were they generally healthy, but they were also a positive bunch of people who rarely, if ever, complained about health issues. Gia's last physical a year ago was "unremarkable," and her physician seemed happy with her exam and lab tests.

Knowing she at least needed some reassurance about her fatigue, she returned to her physician. They did a brief physical exam and ordered some new labs. To her, it seemed quite normal as far as doctor's visits go.

The next week, she had her follow-up visit with the doctor and noticed something about the doctor seemed different. She sat down across from the doctor and asked her, "So how am I?" The doctor was about Gia's age and had been Gia's physician for many years. She said to Gia, "We have the lab results, and I spoke with the pathologist at the lab. Gia, it looks like you have a particular form of leukemia." After she heard the word *leukemia*, the rest of what her doctor said seemed fuzzy and slow. All Gia kept thinking was, "Leukemia—well, that's cancer and I don't have cancer." Her thoughts were spinning.

Gia's doctor knew what was happening. Sadly, this wasn't the first time she had to have this conversation with a patient. She stopped explaining things and said, "Gia. Gia, it's OK, and there is no right or wrong way to react to news like this." At this, her eyes met Gia's, and she saw Gia recognize what was happening. The doctor then slowed down and proceeded to give small bits of information waiting for Gia to take it in. She described the presumed diagnosis, what that could mean, and what tests were next. When she finished, the doctor shook Gia's hand, squeezed her shoulder as she left, and said, "You'll get through this. We will build a team for you, and make sure you bring a support person to your follow-up appointments to take notes."

From that moment on, Gia's life became two separate parts: one was "regular life," which included work, family, and friends; the other was her "new life" as a cancer patient.

Her "new life," that of a "person with cancer" (she specifically chose this terminology instead of "cancer patient"), was a very full life as well. The biopsy she had of her bone marrow (something she would later say is a procedure you should avoid unless you absolutely need it) was followed by more tests and a consultation with an oncologist. Gia kept asking herself, "Why?" Why with such a full life already did she have to add all this?

About two weeks into this new life, she chose a shift in thinking, which she did deliberately. She went from thinking, "What? No, this can't be happening" to "Well, then, 'F-Cancer!' I don't deserve this!" About a day and a half into the "F-Cancer" thinking, she smiled and thought, "Well, I remember Psychology 101 from college and the stages of grief." She seemed to have internalized these stages and thought, "Denial/insulation, anger, bargaining, depression, and acceptance" and then thought, "How I wish those were just a test answer."

As a positive person, her thoughts of "three stages to go" seemed automatic. Then almost immediately, her thoughts gave way to a feeling of overwhelming anger. She just didn't deserve this. Not at all. "Why," "Unfair," and "F-Cancer" just spun through her mind on a continuous loop. She was a good person. She took care of herself, didn't smoke or drink alcohol, exercised, and generally lived a healthy life. "This just isn't fair!" her mind would scream.

As the weeks, doctor visits, rearranging of her life, and all of the other tasks seemingly attached to a cancer diagnosis progressed, she felt like she was passing through a collage of bargaining mixed with depression. This did not match her typical buoyant self, and she knew it. But then she told herself, "You have never had cancer before, have you, Gia?"

As days/weeks passed, Gia began to think a lot about acceptance. She thought, "The rational side of everybody's mind has to accept the reality, right? OK, but to really accept cancer, what does that mean?" So many thoughts; "Do I have to accept this? Don't people who refuse to accept it live longer (or is that a myth)?"

Then she recalled a famous author on a PBS show stating their cancer had "no part in their life." "Wait," she thought, "didn't he have leukemia like me?" And, "I wonder what he died of?"

This internal conversation went on and on.

Gia's second life as a person with cancer continued. There were many details and decisions to consider, such as what to do and what not to do. Her emotions had moved through denial, past anger, and into a mixture of bargaining and depression. She wasn't denying her cancer. She was recognizing it as a reality of her life and admitting to herself that she has a life-altering disease, but she was also facing it with courage. She was not fighting the diagnosis as the author on PBS had. Gia had moved on into acceptance.

At this stage, she realized, "I have control over the *medical* process, to a degree, but what about my internal process?" And then she began to reflect, "What about my thoughts, feelings, emotions, and all that?" So Gia embarked on a journey that day—a journey that changed the course of both of her "lives."

BOB'S STORY

Bob was a powerhouse—successful, wealthy, and all that comes along with that. He was a surgeon and was known as an excellent physician by all. His life had focused on getting to the top of his profession. His family was well cared for financially but completely estranged from him. His children were now all adults and had various levels of contact with him. His ex-wife wanted nothing to do with him. He saw his life as a sacrifice to ensure his family was cared for at any cost. Sadly, the family saw the harder side of all this, something not uncommon for professionals. There was a woman in his life he did consider to be his partner. Bob wasn't a bad guy, but Bob was who he was.

Bob saw his doctor for an annual physical and was good about that process almost every year. He had always been in good health. He exercised, did not drink, and had smoked for five years in college but stopped many years ago. He was conscientious about his diet and tried to live a healthy lifestyle. A year ago, at his physical, his physician said, "Well, Bob, from the looks of your labs, you'll live forever. Must be because you're so mean." His physician said it with a smile, but the whole medical community knew Bob to be demanding, dogmatic, and often just nasty to be around.

During his recent physical, his physician said, "You seem uncomfortable when I palpate," meaning Bob grimaced when the doctor pressed on one spot. Bob simply said, "I think I've been eating too much heavy food."

"Anything else changed, Bob?" the physician asked.

"Well, maybe…" and Bob went on to describe some seemingly odd and random symptoms.

After more physical examination, a blood draw, and some discussing, Bob agreed to get some imaging done on his abdomen. "Better safe than sorry, Bob," said the physician. Bob knew why the imaging was needed.

Bob was back in the doctor's office the next day. (Yes, sometimes for a physician, tests and things can happen quite quickly.) The doctor came in and said, "Well, Bob, you have the 'Big C' based on the scan and labs" (most people knew this as cancer, but his physician thought he was helping break the ice). To be fair, this experienced physician never would have said this to anyone else, but he and Bob had known each other since medical school, and he really didn't know how to break it to him otherwise. So, for better or worse, this is how Bob learned of his cancer diagnosis.

The diagnosis of "probable pancreatic cancer of high stage" dropped on Bob like a bag of cement. Unlike most cancer patients, Bob had lived his adult life as a physician. He knew exactly what this diagnosis meant, and it was not good. Although most people have probably never thought about how they would respond if they received a cancer diagnosis, Bob's career as a physician had told him exactly what he was going to do, at least internally: nothing. Bob had predetermined that he wasn't going to "process" a cancer diagnosis in any mental or emotional way long before he received this diagnosis. Bob would *physically* recognize his cancer. He may receive physical examinations, visit specialists, and allow doctors to perform tests and lab work. But he would not *internally* acknowledge its existence. From an emotional and mental position, there was nothing to work through from his perspective. Bob had seen firsthand pancreatic cancer take lives, and he hated that cancer. "Why couldn't it have just been a massive heart attack?" he thought hopelessly.

We are all different. How each of us processes our diagnosis matters.

Bob and Gia are real people. Of course, their names and some details are altered for privacy, but they are in all aspects real. These patients' stories illustrate two common directions one may take when they face a cancer diagnosis. They appear throughout this book to illustrate two points of view that you may observe and follow when working through your cancer journey. What you can begin to see in their stories is the way each person dealt with their diagnosis and the process we are speaking about.

As you will see as we continue through the book, the way you emotionally and mentally face and process a difficult cancer diagnosis can have a great impact on your own emotional, mental, and even physical well-being. Further, our emotional and mental response to a cancer diagnosis impacts our family and other loved ones, who also have to process what is happening, and their journey is important, too.

At this point of their journeys, the differences between Bob's and Gia's responses may seem small. But as you turn the pages, you will see how those subtle early differences impacted their outcomes tremendously. Gia's initial positivity led her down one path, helped her make better choices, helped her include her family and loved ones in the process, and overall improved her emotional and mental state compared to Bob. Bob never fully accepted his diagnosis. On the outside, some things—such as tests, lab work, and doctor visits—may have increased, but he made no effort at facing his mortality within his own mind and emotions. As you will see, this greatly impacted his decision making, his physical outcomes, and the lives of his loved ones.

Both Bob and Gia experienced many of the same emotions—denial, anger, frustration—but Gia decided to walk *through* the emotions, allowing them to wash over her. She didn't hide and run away; rather, she allowed herself to experience each one as it came, and then she would add in thoughts of positivity. Her process was not easy. There were moments of anger, as you will see. However, because she faced each emotion, she was able to progress through each and into acceptance and increasing empowerment.

Bob, instead, chose to ignore his mental and emotional state. He allowed no time to process his emotions or thoughts. He buried them. Unfortunately, as you will see, Bob never reached acceptance, which impacted him and his family greatly.

YOUR NEXT STEPS

In the Your Next Steps sections at the end of each chapter, I will highlight a few key ways you can apply the concepts we've discussed to your own life. I will keep this as short and to the point as possible. I hope these are beneficial for you. Face your own mortality.

One of the most impactful parts of a cancer diagnosis is facing your own mortality. Yes, some people who have cancer die, but many live. More importantly, your reaction to and evolution through the diagnosis become as helpful as possible and set you up for a successful journey. And although you cannot change the fact of the diagnosis, you can alter the way it affects you.

Is cancer a death sentence? Excellent question. If you look at statistics from international cancer agencies, you see that survival is different based on the type of cancer. For example, at five years, overall survival (including all stages) for breast cancer is 87 percent, but for pancreatic cancer it is 3 percent. Furthermore, the stage at which the cancer is discovered is crucial to survival. The stage of a cancer has to do with how much it has spread upon diagnosis and other factors. A lower stage has less spread and is generally associated with better survival and outcome than a higher stage cancer. Staging is based on a 1 to 4 scale with stage 1 being the least aggressive/invasive and stage 4 the most. As an example, the American Cancer Society lists breast cancer survival at five years at 93 percent for stage 2 and 22 percent for stage 4.

Your physician and healthcare team will help you make sense of all the statistical information. However, it is important to focus on the way YOU see and process the diagnosis. Outside help is excellent for data points and follow-up, but your internal feeling about this life change is crucial. You may choose to see the diagnosis as a statistic, as a wake-up call (i.e., "I've been meaning to look at my health habits"), as confronting your mortality more immediately than many people do, or as an extremely unfair event in your life. Some people experience all of these at once.

But for your health and your life, it is also good to see that the way you process all of this and how you decide to move forward with that process make a difference. It is not easy, but the way you take the journey matters, and your life or the life of a loved one may depend on it.

The diagnosis of cancer is difficult and possibly horrible news, but know that many others have been through this and thrived.

There are many reasons that a life-changing event, such as a cancer diagnosis, is shocking. Although we all realize we will die, for those with this diagnosis, that may be sooner than expected. We are flooded with memories of family, friends, and loved ones who struggled with cancer, and those are often disturbing memories. We wish this was happening to someone else. And on it goes. I am not saying to "Get over it" or "Know you don't have it as bad as others." The message here is that others have been through this before. There is often no positive feeling about it at first, yet embracing this wave of feelings is the first step toward positive movement and empowerment. The rest of this book is dedicated to providing you with perspective and tools for this sometimes uncomfortable but necessary journey to empowerment.

In the next chapter, we will explore how those early decisions by Bob and Gia impacted their next steps, their health, and the emotional and mental well-being of those closest to them. We will continue to follow Bob and Gia through chapter 9.

CHAPTER 2

I HAVE CANCER—I FEEL LOST, ANGRY, CONFUSED, AND SO MUCH MORE

(YOU JUST GOT SOME OF THE WORST NEWS A HUMAN CAN GET; YOU'RE NORMAL)

"Courage is not the absence of fear, but rather the judgment that something else is more important than fear."

—AMBROSE REDMOON

GIA'S NEXT STEPS

At this stage, she realized, "I have control over the medical process, to a degree, but what about my internal process?" And then she began

to reflect, "What about my thoughts, feelings, emotions, and such?" So
Gia embarked on a journey that day—a journey that would change
the course of both her "lives."

Having cancer divided Gia's life into a pre-diagnosis "regular
life" and the totally unwanted "cancer life." She realized this
was the way things were now. She also saw that she held ultimate control over what she thought, how she felt, and how she
processed this new way of being.

She remembered reading about Dr. Viktor Frankl, an Austrian
psychiatrist and Holocaust survivor best known for his 1946
psychological memoir *Man's Search for Meaning*. She decided
that if cancer was bad, then someone who lived through a
concentration camp might have some insights to help get her
out of her angry and obsessive thoughts. She found essays by
Frankl online and saw that he believed meaning came from
three possible sources: purposeful work, love, and courage in
the face of difficulty. He wrote about the "intensification of
inner life" that helped prisoners in the death camps stay alive:

> *Love goes very far beyond the physical person of the beloved. It finds*
> *its deepest meaning in his spiritual being, his inner self. Whether or*
> *not he is actually present, whether or not he is still alive at all, ceases*
> *somehow to be of importance.*

This deep realization also helped Frankl process the death of
his beloved wife in the camps.

Gia knew she wasn't in a "death camp," but she sure did not feel like she was much better off. "People die of cancer," she would think. So she took great comfort that someone who survived a death camp and had real insights could provide her with some legitimate wisdom for her journey.

She read another essay in which Frankl quoted Nietzsche: "He who has a why to live for can bear with almost any how." This somehow struck her heart. Yes, she had circumstances she might not be able to change, but she had control over her mind. She recalled the famous idea Frankl shared of his horrific experience in the camps: "Forces beyond your control can take away everything you possess except one thing: your freedom to choose how you will respond to the situation."

"Well," Gia thought, "it sure feels uncomfortable, but it makes sense. I do have control over how I will respond." This day was a turning point for Gia. It wasn't easy, but it was the start of a new chapter in her journey.

BOB'S NEXT STEPS

The diagnosis of "probable pancreatic cancer of high stage" dropped on Bob like a bag of cement…Bob had predetermined that he wasn't going to "process" a cancer diagnosis in any mental or emotional way long before he received this diagnosis…From an emotional and mental position, there was nothing to work through from his perspective. Bob had seen firsthand pancreatic cancer take lives, and he hated that cancer. *"Why couldn't it have just been a massive heart attack?" he thought hopelessly.*

In contrast to Gia, Bob was not feeling like progressing or being empowered at all. Bob was stunned and grieving the loss of his life before cancer. Bob became more and more angry. He had spent his life telling himself, and those who would listen, that if he ever got cancer, he would likely end it all. "I've seen it close up, and it's horrible. No way would I ever go through that." Bob would recount stories of patients and all the negativity they would experience such as the horrific therapies and side effects. He would go on to say, "If it isn't something curable, it's just not worth living."

It became "put up or shut up" time for Bob. He'd spent a career saying all of this. How was that going to play out in his life now?

His partner asked if he would see a counselor and work through the shock, anger, and disbelief. He flatly said, "No. Furthermore, none of that mind-body BS works anyway." This deepened his anger and at times his rage. Nobody argued with him that this was an easy diagnosis, or massively life changing, or about any detail. His partner simply wished he didn't have to add the mental suffering he was creating on top of everything else.

THE STAGES OF GRIEF/PROCESSING: ARE THEY REAL AND DO THEY MATTER?

As you can see, the differences between Bob and Gia are unfolding as two opposite methods of coping and processing. Gia is not "happy" with her cancer diagnosis but is open to learning a better way. Bob is ruled by his anger and grief and is not open to learning.

Gia received the news of her cancer as most people do—with surprise and shock. Her initial thoughts were not "constructive," but they were normal. What she did at first was to make sense of what she was thinking and feeling and then work toward a solution focus rather than a fear or anger focus. Was this easy? No. No, it was not. I watched it happen. The important thing is that it did happen.

Upon diagnosis, Bob had the same amount of surprise and shock as Gia. He was, like any human, completely entitled to those thoughts and feelings. He chose to take the step to more anger and agitation.

As I will mention elsewhere in the book, Bob, like anyone else, is entitled to react and do as he please. It is a human right, and I would never attempt to deny him. So I am not judging him or his reaction but rather using it in a clinical sense as a counterpoint to what I have seen as more helpful strategies in moving toward empowerment.

Most people have heard of the stages of grief originally written by Elisabeth Kübler-Ross, which include denial, anger, bargaining, depression, and acceptance. These stages were developed to describe the process patients go through as they come to terms with their terminal illness.

Although there is some debate about the accuracy of these stages in all people, I can certainly tell you from years of working with patients during some of the hardest moments of their life, the stages of grief are excellent observations.

These are common stages that both patients and loved ones go through. What I have seen, and many people relate to, is that a person often gets "stuck" in a stage and, once stuck, has a great deal of difficulty progressing.

Nobody (or very few people) would argue that a person diagnosed with cancer should not feel these things. That is the human condition. And it stands to reason that as we are all individuals, we may experience a stage or two more or less intensely than another. The important aspect is that we continue to move through these completely valid feelings and stages to arrive at a point that affords us maximum health and benefit as we (or our loved ones) live with our cancer journey.

YOUR NEXT STEPS

Here are some factors I have seen that make the realization and processing of the grieving stages work toward better outcomes and eventually lead to empowerment.

Recognizing the stages are real.

- Honor them. They are normal and not a sign of human frailty. You are wired to process large shocks this way.
- We may choose different words to describe the phases of this process, but most people go through them in the same order. However, you may process them in a different order or move rapidly through one and not the other. As I will discuss later in the book, there can be "cycles" or "grief within grief," all of which is completely normal.
- Based on our individual past experiences, personality, and other factors, we all process the diagnosis and every other part of cancer at varying speeds. Some people experience more denial while others experience more anger. There is no right or wrong way to process. The important thing is to let the process happen. Although there are predictable steps in the process, you may know where you will take longer to process (or it may surprise you). This book provides insight as to where you may need help, support, and personal growth.

Know that however you move through them, it is YOUR way.

- Moving, processing, and growing are the important parts. You will not do this like others, and that is perfectly normal.

Know that close supporters and loved ones are going through their version of this as well.

- Those around us may not realize this will happen. Often, they know they have shock and sadness but do not realize they have to process the entire diagnosis, change in life, and relationships as well. This often helps you, the patient, to understand others' reactions as well as to help or suggest help for them.

Realize that acceptance is not resignation.

- The act of acceptance is embracing the reality of the journey and all it encompasses while also knowing that you have control over your responses to and interpretation of the process. Acceptance allows you to reset and move on to an empowered, proactive, and progressive state, which, in my experience, is healthier and associated with better outcomes throughout the journey.

Find outside help if you cannot process through a stage, need help understanding a loved one's processes, or feel lost in your own process.

- For flow and simplicity, I will use the term *counselor* throughout the book to represent whatever form of outside help you choose. You may find a psychiatrist, psychologist, counselor, spiritual advisor, or one of the many other helpers to facilitate your journey. The important thing is that you resonate with them and that they resonate with you. As a note, you may already have a relationship with a counselor. If not, know that the process of finding the right person takes time. Ask friends or professionals for referrals (your healthcare team will likely have many), and work with someone you feel you resonate with.

CHAPTER 3

HOW AM I SUPPOSED TO FEEL AND THINK?

DOES IT REALLY MAKE A DIFFERENCE?

"Cancer is a word, not a sentence."

—JOHN DIAMOND

GIA'S NEXT STEPS

"Well," Gia thought, "it sure feels uncomfortable, but it makes sense. I do have control over how I will respond." This day was a turning point for Gia. It wasn't easy, but it was the start of a new chapter in her journey.

Gia had been through what seemed like another lifetime since her diagnosis. Dealing with her "two lives" was time consuming, and there were mornings she would wake up feeling like maybe it was all a dream. It wasn't.

As she made the turning point in coming to grips with being on this cancer journey, she worked hard to find better ways of thinking, feeling, and relating to her diagnosis, the changes in her body, and her new "other" life. She read anything that seemed related. She kept a journal and tried to log her insights. She watched online content of all kinds, challenged lifelong thought patterns and beliefs she had held—trying anything she thought may help her process.

Was every day a triumph? No. But every day, as hard as some were, was a chance to make a choice to control the one thing she could—her response to cancer being in her life. Her counselor encouraged her and would say, "It's not easy, Gia, but it is worth it." Even on the days where her treatment wore her out or the medication she took for the side effects of therapy seemed as bad as the therapy itself, Gia knew it was true. On those days, she gave herself a break and did what she could.

Gia would reset her mind every morning. She had no control ultimately over a lot of the details. She would stop before the day unfolded and be grateful for whatever she could, be open to learning new lessons, and remain positive and hopeful for any blessings the day may have. Astonishingly, in the beginning, she found something to be grateful for every day.

BOB'S NEXT STEPS

His partner asked if he would see a counselor and work through the shock, anger, and disbelief. He flatly said, "No. Furthermore, none of that mind-body BS works anyway." This deepened his anger and at times his rage. Nobody argued it was an easy diagnosis...His loved ones simply wished he didn't have to add the mental suffering he was creating on top of everything else.

As Bob and his attitude seemed to darken with each day, his partner became worried—and for good reason. He was more withdrawn and angrier than normal. He didn't seem depressed but just holding on to anger at his core. He seemed to visibly age, daily.

Bob refused any outside help for his feelings, mind, emotions, or any other "touchy-feely" aspects of his cancer diagnosis. He would say things such as, "I'm not negative. I'm a realist"; or "None of that counseling BS works"; or "I've got one of the worst cancers you can have. What do you expect me to think?"

Bob had hit the "anger" stage and was not letting go. He was mad, and "Damn, he had a right to be." He knew all about the so-called stages of grief, and he didn't "buy that BS either." When asked, he would reply, "It's still my life, and I'll do what I like with it."

HOW OUR DIFFERENCES PLAY OUT

Bob and Gia certainly had a divergence in their approach to processing cancer in their lives. One thing I have seen patients struggle with over the years is a realistic set of concerns related to how one processes a cancer diagnosis. "What is the point, and does it matter anyway?" is a common and completely legitimate thought.

In Bob's case, he took the "What is the point, and does it matter?" thought to the extreme of "There is no point, and it does not matter or help." He was angry and resistant to any alternative thoughts or ways of processing. As I mentioned before, this is his right, and he decided to stay in a mental and emotional place where he was a victim to all circumstances.

Gia, on the other hand, had no less of an emotional crisis facing this question. The difference is that she decided, regardless of how it all seemed, to focus on what she could control. She reset her mind daily to the "What do I have control over?" outlook and practiced gratitude daily.

Getting stuck in one of the stages of grief (denial, anger, bargaining, depression, and acceptance/empowerment) is easy to do—almost as easy as trying to skip one. For most of us, it is natural to get stuck. It is human nature. Therefore, having someone to offer outside, objective, and professional help is crucial.

In all the patient experiences I have witnessed and participated in, one thing is certain: although we are all different, the process is similar among us and should lead to a healthier relationship with your diagnosis. And it really does make a difference.

You may wonder if there is any research or science that has looked at the connection between what we think and the way it affects our cancer journey. Actually, there is. In a 2015 scientific publication, authors looked at the basic factors of this question and came to the following conclusions:

> The quality of life of cancer survivors is multifaceted and is influenced by a variety of cancer-related and non-cancer factors from the time of cancer diagnosis through long-term survivorship. Physical health and symptoms directly affect mental health, and vice versa. Cancer outcomes—like those of most illnesses—are influenced by socioeconomic status, access to care, supportive services, and rural-urban factors, all of which contribute to the well-being of cancer survivors in North Carolina.
>
> Screening for mental health morbidity is just as important as monitoring physical health among cancer survivors, and mental health screening needs to be better integrated into active cancer treatment and survivorship. ("Physical and Mental Health among Cancer Survivors: Considerations for Long-Term Care and Quality of Life," by Michelle J. Naughton and Kathryn E. Weaver [PMID: 25046097].)

The importance of this, and some of the other scientific papers I refer to, is that there are scientific investigations into these factors and that they match real-life patient experiences I have witnessed. This paper shows that the way cancer physically affects us, the environment surrounding us, and how we interact and interpret those factors do affect our cancer journey.

In 2016, different authors looked specifically at the roles of emotion in breast cancer survival. They evaluated the emotional personal toll of the diagnosis as well as the connections between emotion, stress, and survival physiologically. A few of their conclusions:

> In conclusion, there is still much to learn about the nature of the relationship between emotion, regulation, and adaptation to breast cancer. However, it is clear that effective regulatory processes merit significant consideration in both research and clinical practice, due to their intervening role between stress and health outcomes. Further research on emotion regulation may help women with breast cancer better manage the emotional challenges associated with diagnosis and treatment. ("Emotions and Emotion Regulation in Breast Cancer Survivorship," by Claire C. Conley, Brenden T. Bishop, and Barbara L. Andersen [PMID: 27517969].)

There are many other research papers, books, and expert opinions on this topic. I mention these as examples. Even though the scientific community may not agree on the extent of influence our emotions, thought life, and related factors have on the cancer journey, they generally do agree it has influence.

In plain terms, "science" as we see in publications agrees with what most people who have been through this cancer journey would tell you: the emotional, mental, and "internal" journey as you go through the process is intimately related to the physical, medical, and cancer outcome portion of your journey.

YOUR NEXT STEPS

The Six OKs

1. It's OK that it is a process.

As a child, when I was most frustrated with some project, my father would say, "Rome wasn't built in a day," which was the last thing I thought I wanted to hear. Most of us "know" this. However, in the midst of a process, it can be anything but comforting to hear. The fact is that no one "arrives" immediately. That would be nonhuman. What I am saying is that it is not a destination; it is a process. In some cases, this can be a reason why people get depressed and feel like giving in or giving up. The important thing is to realize that every day you'll have a piece of this process to work on, and that is something you do control.

2. It's OK to go at your own pace.

Just as most people understand the idea that this all is a "process," they also realize that each person moves at different speeds. You may be more skilled in some areas than others. We all are. But those areas are different for each one of us and depend on our personality, experience, and other factors. Your skill and experience in an area may make parts of that process faster or slower for you. Realizing that the journey to empowerment is a process and not a destination can be frustrating. Additionally, realizing that you take more time to move through a stage compared to another person may cause you to feel like giving up. However, most people find that once they realize this difference and let go of their idea of a schedule that needs to be met, they begin to feel much freer and more relaxed to move forward.

3. It's OK to take longer in one area than another.

We all move at different speeds through the process, and we may take longer in one area compared to other areas. Remember, it isn't a race or a competition. As mentioned above, you have unique experiences and backgrounds, so your time and depth of process required at each step will be yours. Denial may be easier to move through than anger for one person, and the opposite will be true for another. It's your process, and the goal is healing, peace, and empowerment.

4. It's OK to go back and relive a stage.

The idea of processing a stage as a "one and done" is a nice idea but rarely realistic. We all have things we think we have processed and then someone calls us, someone says something, we see a photo, or any number of triggers, and we realize we were not as "done" with that stage as we thought. This is fine, and it's completely normal. Expect the unexpected and know that it means positive forward motion when it happens. Humans are deep beings, and it takes time to honor our depth.

5. It's OK to have bad days.

Some days, you'll just be over it. Personal growth, empowerment, and so forth will all seem like the worst endeavor anyone ever suggested. That's fine. It's normal. It's human. Take a day to let things just be, a moment to refocus and rest. Prior to cancer being part of your life, you had bad days. You will now. It's OK. It's a reason to pause, rest, and regroup.

6. It's OK to want to give up.

Every human, even the seemingly most driven and focused, have times they want to give up. This is normal. In the same way, it is OK to have a bad day and rest rather than quit. It is also OK to have the overwhelming feeling of wanting to quit. Being aware that it is coming, and that it is normal and part of the process, gives you power over the feeling. Do what you need to do to regroup, get outside perspective, and rest. The feeling doesn't last forever; it just seems like it will at the time.

So everything is "OK" for me; what does that mean?

The point is that our thought process and attitude make a difference, and in the long run, it is best to stick with your process and do your best to avoid getting stuck. So if it does make a difference, is there a roadmap to help me? Yes. I will use a great deal of experience, the prevailing scientific literature, common sense, and realism to provide a way for you to navigate it all.

CHAPTER 4

IS THERE A PROCESS I CAN USE TO MAKE SENSE OF THIS?

WHAT'S THE PATH TO MOVE ME FROM WHERE I AM TO A MORE STABLE, WORKABLE PLACE?

"The ultimate measure of a man is not where he stands in moments of comfort and convenience, but where he stands at a time of challenge and controversy."

—DR. MARTIN LUTHER KING JR.

GIA'S NEXT STEPS

Gia would reset her mind every morning. She had no control ulti-mately over a lot of the details. She would stop before the day unfolded and be grateful for whatever she could, be open to learning new les-

sons, and positive and hopeful for any blessings the day may have.
Astonishingly, in the beginning, she found something to be grateful
for every day.

As Gia worked with her counselor, journaled, thought, challenged, and processed, she slowly started to gain a sense of some control over her response to her situation as well as her overall emotional state. Despite the reality of cancer, she began to feel that she had a better outlook and even felt better physically.

BOB'S NEXT STEPS

Bob had hit the "anger" stage and was not letting go. He was mad, and
"Damn, he had a right to be." He knew all about the so-called stages of
grief, and he didn't "buy that BS either." When asked, he would reply,
"It's still my life, and I'll do what I like with it."

Bob was not really "working through" much. He resented the cancer, the bleak outlook, and was mourning the loss of his life even before he actually died. Each day, he became more and more angry and insulated from his partner. His doctor friends offered help, and he simply refused. The likelihood of any therapies working for his cancer, as advanced as it was, statistically was very low. He opted to only receive palliative/symptomatic and comfort care if he needed it. He quickly sold his practice to an associate and retired.

As he left medical practice, he retired to a dark angry place in his home. His partner avoided him. He drank heavily and would lash out when people offered comfort.

THE PROCESS

We all have control over the choices we make in life and how we deal with unpleasant and life-altering news. Bob and Gia continued down two different paths. Since you are still reading this book, I assume you want to explore a better roadmap—one that leads to a process more like Gia's rather than Bob's.

Bob let his anger and frustration with his world-changing cancer diagnosis send him to a dark and isolated place. His prior thoughts about not getting counseling for anything in his life seemed to intensify after knowing he had cancer. Again, this was his choice to make, but it led him away from peace and empowerment.

Gia was not any happier to be diagnosed with cancer than Bob, but she realized she could control some things, and her thoughts and ability to be in charge of many areas of her life motivated her to do the work and stay on the journey. It didn't come naturally for her, but she just kept taking baby steps and doing what she could to process and seek help. The more she did, the more rewarding she saw the process.

In this chapter, we will look at the general pathway components to a process of acceptance, empowerment, and maximal emotional mastery over your own cancer journey. In the next chapter, we will discuss specific areas that may be different for you versus others and how to customize the information to fit your needs.

Keep in mind that when I use the term *process* or *cancer journey*, I mean that process or journey specific to you as either the person who has cancer or the person loving, caring for, and supporting the person with cancer. Regardless of which category you are in (the patient or the support person), the first step in a path toward acceptance and empowerment is *assessment*.

SELF-ASSESSMENT: WHAT "STAGE" ARE YOU IN?

Remember, these stages are all completely normal. Looking at your progress and remembering everyone goes through the stages differently is crucial. Once you know where you are starting, you can plot a course to an empowered path. Ask yourself, be honest, and consider asking a trusted friend if needed if you are in denial, anger, bargaining, depression, or acceptance.

IT IS FINE TO BE WHERE YOU ARE, YOUR BRAIN NEEDS IT

Although people may disagree over specifics about the stages of grief, most agree that the stages are a reasonable process the human mind uses to move through shock (such as a cancer diagnosis) to a healthier place (acceptance and empowerment). So, much like a baby learning to crawl before walking, you need to do whatever your brain needs to facilitate this process. If you are still in denial, that is normal; if you are in bargaining, that is fine, too. The point is to move through these stages in a healthy manner and allow your brain and emotions to progress.

Remember, everyone has a different speed. Just as we typically need to work through the stages in some type of order for our brain to process, we all have variable speeds in which we work. Regardless of your process speed (or phase), the most important factor is that it happens. There is no benefit to getting stuck.

Just as assessment is crucial to moving through to the acceptance stage of grief, it's also important to understand that some seemingly odd questions may pop into your mind. Here are two questions that are worth considering.

How Can I Move Forward (It Feels Good to Be ____—Mad, Sad...)?

Although verbalized less often, this is an extremely common question. This, again, is a normal thought. You have a variety of feelings throughout the process and not all feelings are good. For example, when you are angry, it can feel good (and rewarding) to be mad. After all, you do have cancer! This is normal and healthy to a point. When this helps you process the stage you are in, it is fine. When it becomes a reason for you to become stuck, it is unhealthy. This is one reason getting some outside help to facilitate the processing can be crucial.

When I'm Done with a Stage, Am I Really "Done"?

Yes and no. In one sense, the processing part of that stage has passed, and you are unlikely to circle back to a stage in its full form. But being human, it is completely normal to have any emotion recycle and hit you seemingly from nowhere. Denial, anger, or any of the other stages can reappear at any time. This may mean you need to spend a bit more time processing, or it may mean it is your brain working on moving forward. This is an excellent thing to address with your counselor.

HOW YOUR "TRUE NORTH" CAN HELP YOU PROGRESS THROUGH THE STAGES OF GRIEF

We all need a reason to progress and change. Processing the diagnosis of cancer and all it entails is no different. However, it requires a much bigger motivator. For example, Gia did it for herself, her health, and for some internal belief that it was the right thing. Bob did not, and he stayed angry. I have had mothers do it for their family, partners do it for their relationship goals, and many other reasons. It is not an easy task, and yet it is crucial to your health. Finding a "true north" to focus on is critical. We all get lost, stall out, get discouraged, and confront other derailing events. Having a place to reset our focus is critical to our success. My colleague, Dr. Samantha Brody, authored the book *Overcoming Overwhelm* (Sounds True Publishing, 2019) where she lays out a step-by-step plan to get from overwhelm to moving forward. She says that one key is locating your "true north." I strongly recommend this book, and there will be information about it in the resources section at the end of this book.

YOUR NEXT STEPS

Realize that it is OK to indulge the "it feels good to be ___" perspective.

We are all human, and sometimes feeling negative emotions (sad, angry, depressed, etc.) does "feel good." But just like realizing you will want to quit the journey toward empowerment is freeing and provides you with a tool to continue moving forward, so does knowing that "it feels good to feel bad" is a short-term and fleeting feeling. Acknowledge it and move forward.

Find ways to become centered in the storm.

Fun, easy, or exciting may not be things a person would say about this process because for many people, at least in the beginning, it does not seem like those apply. Once again, this is normal. We all need the grace to be human and the realization that there are ways to move forward. Although taking stock of you and your life can be difficult, finding your "true north" and a place to reset on both good and bad days is crucial to your process and your journey toward empowerment.

As I conclude this chapter, I want you to know that you can do this. There is a process, and it is healthy to start where you are. The entire journey may be challenging, but it is possible and beneficial for you to see it simply as a part of your cancer journey. While there may be common threads within the process, you need to do your work. Your journey is your own to walk, and you must walk it.

CHAPTER 5

WHAT IS UNIQUE TO ME, AND WHAT IS COMMON TO EVERYONE?

ALTHOUGH THE PROCESS IS SIMILAR, WHO YOU ARE MAKES IT UNIQUE!

"You gain strength, courage, and confidence by every experience in which you really stop to look fear in the face. You must do the thing which you think you cannot do."

—ELEANOR ROOSEVELT

GIA'S NEXT STEPS

As Gia worked with her counselor, journaled, thought, challenged, and processed, she slowly started to gain a sense of some control over her response to her situation as well as her overall emotional state. Despite the reality of cancer, she began to feel that she had a better outlook and even felt better physically.

As Gia did the rewarding, but at times difficult, work of moving to empowerment, she realized she had some things she experienced that were different from what her counselor mentioned. She also had seemingly different experiences in depth or timing from the books and online materials she looked at. She spoke to her counselor about this and the reply was, "Well, of course, Gia, you are going to go through this in your way." Gia found this comforting.

BOB'S NEXT STEPS

As he left medical practice, he retired to a dark angry place in his home. His partner avoided him. He drank heavily and would lash out when people offered comfort.

Bob wasn't into processing, achieving empowerment, or anything positive. He felt righteous anger, and he held on to that. He was mourning his "death sentence" and the loss of the life he had planned.

WE ARE ALL IN CHARGE OF AND RESPONSIBLE FOR OUR LIVES AND THIS PROCESS

I want to make a critical point here. Although many may disagree with Bob and his way of dealing with the situation, it is important that we understand this was his decision. In the end, with a cancer (or any) diagnosis, the decision as to how we process it is completely our own. It is often disturbing to those around us, but we are indeed in charge of our lives and decisions about our response to the diagnosis.

It is likely that Bob would not be the typical reader of this book. In fact, when I spoke to him about these ideas, he got so angry that I thought he'd have a heart attack in my office. Although it is difficult to let people "go their own way" (even when we have encouraged them otherwise), it is important to let go of the outcome you desire for them.

As you now see, Gia chose a different path than Bob and worked diligently. Even when she did not really want to, she moved through and did the hard work of self-discovery. Although she would often say that the process did not get easier, she would also say that it got to be more rewarding as she moved forward. She certainly did things her way, and that is the only way to do it.

In looking at your own specific needs and your pathway through this process, you should consider your own personality, how you normally deal with unpleasant news, and your other personality traits. One concept is universal: if it isn't all yours and you don't own it, the process won't work at a deep level. In other words, you, and only you, can walk through this. Certainly, you have support around you, but if you do not make the walk (and work) your own, it will be easy to drift into denial and stay there.

This is the juncture where many ask, "What is the point? I'm fatigued. These cancer therapies have taken over my life, and I have all sorts of side effects. Is my mental and emotional processing that important?" As you have seen from Bob's story, he did not see a point and stayed in his original mindset. This was still a fight for Gia almost daily, but it often fueled her desire to work on the process.

Keeping in mind it is your decision and the way you approach it is all yours, in my experience, the way you process does make a great deal of difference. If you choose to claim ownership of this process by developing your mental and emotional health around your cancer journey, it will have its challenging moments. But with those challenges come empowerment. You will find that regardless of the physical cancer outcome, your life and your journey with cancer reaches far beyond the cancer itself. This book is dedicated to guiding you to that empowerment and the healing it can affect for the "whole you"—physical, mental, emotional, and all that you are.

A common and very realistic question I hear is, "But if I'm going to die anyway, isn't it pointless to go through all of this?" In my many years of working with patients on their personal cancer journey, I can honestly say that of all the factors that affect one's outcome (for better or worse), choosing to embrace the empowerment of their mental and emotional work is the most significant. I have seen firsthand the effect it has on the outcome of the individual as well as their family and loved ones. Yes, people with cancer die. But many live. If you want to really enhance your positive possibilities, my suggestion is that you should. Because my observation is that it is worth it.

WHAT DOES MODERN SCIENCE SAY ABOUT EMPOWERMENT?

The term *empowerment* is common. The point of this book is to show anyone dealing with cancer that moving to a place from victimhood toward empowerment is both mentally and physically helpful. The idea of empowerment is not just a pop psychology construct. Below are some quotes from scientific research and writing on the topic of empowerment in cancer patients.

An excellent review published in 2019 concluded:

> Unlike traditional approaches to empowerment, patient's expression of empowerment does not mainly reside in the direct control of their condition as much as in an active role within the relationship with caretakers, such as the ability to choose the doctor, the care team, or the health organization in charge of their healthcare. Emerging aspects from this analysis of patient's perspective are central in order to adequately consider empowerment in the care process and to provide more effective care strategies. ("The Patient

Perspective: Investigating Patient Empowerment Enablers and Barriers within the Oncological Care Process," by Luca Bailo, Paolo Guiddi, and Giulia Marton [PMID: 31123495].)

In a review of patient empowerment, research authors concluded that a multitude of factors went into the formation of an empowered patient:

> The thematic synthesis of the papers resulted in seven analytical themes being identified: empowerment as an ongoing process, knowledge is power, having an active role, communication and interaction between patients and health care professionals, support from being in a group, religion and spirituality, and gender. ("What Facilitates 'Patient Empowerment'" in Cancer Patients during Follow-Up: A Qualitative Systematic Review of the Literature," by C. R. Jørgensen and associates [PMID: 28758544].)

And regarding one of the most difficult-to-manage portions of cancer care—pain—authors concluded:

> On the basis of these findings, we propose a conceptual model to empower patients in controlling cancer pain. We recommend focusing on pain treatment given by the professional, on the active involvement of the patient, and on the interaction of both. Our model might also be useful for other patient groups or specific contexts, especially in symptom management. ("Patient Empowerment in Cancer Pain Management: An Integrative Literature Review," by N. TeBoveldt and associates [PMID: 24816749].)

As mentioned above, there are many scientific papers on the phenomenon and importance of empowerment in medicine, specifically cancer care. The purpose of placing these excerpts here is to give a brief overview of that research.

YOUR NEXT STEPS

Realize that the idea of empowerment is a real, scientifically verified factor in your healing journey. After all, I would not have the word in the title of the book were it not just that important.

As mentioned before, be OK with this being about you, about your process and your timing. You will not do this the same way as any other person, and that is both appropriate and necessary.

If the nagging questions "What's the point?" and "Is it worth it?" arise (as they will), remember that it's about you and your healing. Ultimately, the point is you and your quality of life. Only you know if anything is "worth it." But if you have read this far, I'm betting you feel it is. If you need a second opinion, I believe you are "worth it," as you deserve the best inner process and healing. You are "the point."

In summary, remember that it all must be about you because your mind, body, and spirit will only respond to you being real with yourself. You need to process and progress as your body and mind dictate. For some, this focus on self or self-care may feel uncomfortable, but you need to do it. We are often raised not to be selfish. Self-care is not a selfish act. As the saying goes, "You cannot pour from an empty cup." We also cannot heal if we have no resources.

If you are ready to move forward and want to look more deeply into a specific area, the resources at the end of the book will help.

At this point, you may be thinking, "OK, I'm working on me; what about everyone else I know?" Ah, yes. Other humans. Just when we try to get ourselves together, we talk to someone else (and that can be where real self-development begins).

CHAPTER 6

FAMILY AND FRIENDS—HOW DO I INVOLVE THEM IN A HEALTHY WAY?

THE PEOPLE YOU SURROUND YOURSELF WITH ARE A CRUCIAL COMPONENT TO YOUR HEALTH

"If you think you are enlightened, go and spend a week with your family."

—RAM DASS

GIA'S NEXT STEPS

As Gia did the rewarding, but at times difficult, work of moving to empowerment, she realized she had some things she experienced

that were different from what her counselor mentioned. She also had
seemingly different experiences in depth or timing from the books and
online materials she looked at. She spoke to her counselor about this
and the reply was, "Well, of course, Gia, you are going to go through
this in your way." Gia found this comforting.

One area where Gia was struggling was with her family relationships. Although she was single, both of her parents were
alive, and she had a brother whom she was close to. She also
had a small, but close, network of friends that she had known
for five or more years each. Of course, their responses were
highly varied. Some were worse off than Gia seemed to be,
some distant, and some unsure what to do. Most were pretty
good about boundaries, but the variety of emotions they held
were overwhelming.

She did have to tell a few that she needed a little space. For
some, she recommended counseling as it had helped her. One
individual became so negative that Gia had to dig deep to
resolve the core issues that permeated their relationship. She
wasn't sure how much interpersonal toxicity and negativity
played into her newfound mental emotional journey, as she
discovered in this relationship, but she assumed it wasn't helpful.

Although her family and friends meant well, Gia was inundated
with advice, articles, doctor recommendations, and websites
with information ranging from fasting to celery juice detox,
brushing therapies, and many other interesting ideas. The

people who care about us want nothing more than to help, but if she did everything they offered, she would be busy every minute of every day.

BOB'S NEXT STEPS

Bob wasn't into processing, achieving empowerment, or anything positive. He felt righteous anger, and he held on to that. He was mourning his "death sentence" and the loss of the life he had planned... Although many may disagree with Bob and his way of dealing with the situation, it is important that we see this was his decision. In the end, with a cancer (or any) diagnosis, the decision as to how we process it is completely our own.

Bob's experience with family and friends was just about the opposite of Gia's. He was so closed off that they found him impossible to deal with. Some let go. Some became very distraught over everything because it seemed like they had more invested in Bob "trying" than he did.

A well-meaning family member even set an appointment with a local respected integrative oncologist for a second opinion. Bob was angry, but it was a favorite niece who arranged this. Even though he went, it ended poorly.

FAMILY AND EXTERNAL INFLUENCES: MEDICINE OR POISON?

Obviously, we are seeing Bob and Gia trending in quite different directions. Although we all have individual choice and self-determination, I am writing to those who would hopefully choose to approach the journey more like Gia than Bob. So what is the root of their differences?

Bob withdrew more, and it showed. If he did anything the family asked, it was done begrudgingly and with anger. In my personal conversations with him, this was because he honestly believed there was no point, and he believed time spent getting other opinions and seeking connection were just a waste of the time he had left. Bob created distance and boundaries by his behavior and attitude. People literally left him alone. That served his purpose.

Gia, on the other hand, was working on herself diligently and realizing that family and friends were both a great help and a hindrance. Most were completely well meaning, and she knew that. Some were maybe too aggressive in trying to help, and some were awkward in relating to her due to their own issues. She understood most of this. Gia wanted support and interaction but needed space from those who were too helpful or too negative in her life. These were difficult conversations, but they were respected by all she spoke to and gave her the balance of connection and space she needed.

Your cancer diagnosis and journey can overtake your whole

world. Up to this point, we have focused on you and helping you get your journey to a level of empowerment. But what about those around you? Do they affect you? How does your diagnosis and journey affect them? Can they ultimately move you toward or away from empowerment? How do you navigate this often-sensitive terrain?

An excellent scientific review outlines what most people would guess—cancer affects everyone around us:

> Results from multilevel models indicated that family functioning was important. Families that were able to act openly, express feelings directly, and solve problems effectively had lower levels of depression. Direct communication of information within the family was associated with lower levels of anxiety. Aside from differences in anxiety due to cancer type, patients' illness characteristics appear to be risk factors in patients' but not relatives' depression and anxiety. The results from the current study suggest that researchers and clinicians need to be family-focused as cancer affects the whole family, not just the patient. ("The Psychological Impact of a Cancer Diagnosis on Families: The Influence of Family Functioning and Patients' Illness Characteristics on Depression and Anxiety," by B. Edwards and V. Clarke [PMID: 15295777].)

Your family and friends can be neutral, a healing force, or toxic. It happens that some will change after the shock of the diagnosis wears off, and this can be for better or worse. It is important to know that this is all normal and based on their "stuff" and not you.

Below are some specific ideas for this tricky area.

FRIENDS AND FAMILY GO THROUGH THE SAME STAGES

Although the experience is slightly different, a person who cares for you will have their own version of denial, anger, bargaining, depression, and acceptance. In some ways, it is harder when it is NOT you, as you have no control over their process, and you love and care for this person on the cancer journey.

Frankly, sometimes your loved ones are more of a wreck than you are. Although we may have to limit or eliminate some of those within our circle, they also need a break. They received bad, life-altering news as well.

THE PEOPLE YOU SURROUND YOURSELF WITH ON THE JOURNEY ARE CRUCIAL

To some, this makes complete sense. To others, it seems an overstatement. There is no way to overstate this factor in your health. This is a fight for your quality and quantity of life; for you, this is the paramount and singular priority. Therefore, who you surround yourself with is crucial, as they will be the ones speaking into your life most often, offering help, and being the most available for you to ask for help. Toxic people, bad relationships, and other negative influences cannot be tolerated in your world.

YOU CAN LEAD THEM THROUGH THE PROCESS

Something we can forget is that living with cancer doesn't make you helpless. If you choose to do the empowering mental and emotional work, you can lead your loved ones through the process, too. It may seem odd, but as the person with cancer, you have more control than they do, and they look to you for cues. It is not your responsibility to change them, but people with cancer often forget the power they have.

This may be easier than assessing yourself since you know these people and their patterns, thought processes, and so forth. With likely a few exceptions, you basically know how they will all respond. Be open to being wrong, but factor this knowledge into your planning when interacting with them.

Use positive statements. Model the behavior you want them to exhibit. If they are trying but get off track, a gentle reminder is often enough to help. Keep in mind, they may be stuck in denial, anger, or another stage; honor that. You may need to let them know you understand but need to have space from them while they process.

WHAT IF THEY ARE STUCK IN NEGATIVITY AND ARE POISONING YOU?

Usually, except for people you live with, it is difficult, but appropriate, for you to distance yourself from people at times. As I mentioned, this is about you and your life, literally. You decide what and who you allow in your life. For individuals who please people and strive for "happiness for all," this is enormously difficult. Think of it this way: if you were sick and there was a pill that could help or cure you, would you toss it out and not take it? Allowing personal relationships to poison you and your process is just like not taking the pill.

WHAT IF IT IS YOUR SPOUSE, PARTNER, OR A CHILD WHO LIVES WITH YOU?

This can be one of the most difficult issues, if not the most difficult, in this area to address. People you live with, and cannot easily distance yourself from, can be the most healing force or the most continuous poison you can be exposed to. In almost all cases, we certainly want to maintain our primary family relationships. Although there are times I have seen cutting a family member off or leaving them become necessary, it is generally not the most desired pathway. I would modify this, however, if someone is in an abusive relationship. I only see people deteriorate and die faster in abusive relationships. In those cases, leaving is preferable and healthier. But let's assume it isn't a worst-case scenario. Then all the above advice applies. Remember, they are in shock, grieving, and traumatized. Give them space and grace.

IT'S IMPORTANT TO KEEP OPEN COMMUNICATION

Be loving but honest. If they need time and space, great. Continue to check in with one another. If you need support, ask them to help you the best way they can. It can be one of the most difficult things to do. The closer the relationship, the more up front and firmer you must be. And please, get outside help (counseling, etc.) for the sake of the relationship(s) and all concerned.

Can you have difficult conversations with them? You love and care about these people. Being honest about their influence and its effect on you may be some of the hardest conversations you'll have and one of the hardest things to do—in most cases, more difficult than your own self-assessment.

YOUR NEXT STEPS

Remember that you and your health are more important than anything.

You cannot take second place to anyone. This may seem selfish and heartless to some, but this is your life. Understand that the people around you and their energy and influence are as strong (or stronger) than any medicine.

Have the hard conversations.

The ease or difficulty of a frank and open conversation will largely depend on your current relationship, level of autonomy, and other factors. The bottom line is that the conversation needs to happen. Initially, it can be electronic with many people. For example, a private message saying you need a little time to process (before getting together, talking, going out, etc.) can be helpful. Of course, the more you are concerned about the person and their influence, the more difficult it may be. Be loving but firm; this is your life. Here's a tip: use "I" statements (e.g., "I need to be sure I'm hearing helpful ideas," "I need some space," etc.). Remember that they are processing their own grief and are likely at a different stage than you. They may not be to acceptance and empowerment yet. Whatever you do, be consistent and persistent.

You must act.

Not acting is like taking poison daily; it is not going to help you. Act. If necessary, get counseling together with someone.

In summary, those you love and are surrounded by are a huge factor in your process and can be "medicine or poison." Although you may not be able to avoid friends and family and their reactions, you can manage it all. It may seem unfair, but it is critical you take responsibility for and control of these relationships. Remember, this is not about being selfish; this is literally about your health and your life.

At this point, you are likely thinking, "I get that this book is about navigating the inner journey during my cancer diagnosis, but what is the external journey like and how does that connect to the internal one?" It would be unrealistic to not mention the external experience but more importantly where it overlaps with your inner journey.

CHAPTER 7

ARE THERE STEPS IN THE "EXTERNAL" CANCER JOURNEY?

HOW DO THEY RELATE TO WHAT I'M WORKING ON HERE?

"Time is shortening. But every day that I challenge this cancer and survive is a victory for me."

—INGRID BERGMAN

GIA'S NEXT STEPS

Although her family and friends meant well, Gia was inundated with advice, articles, doctor recommendations, and websites with information ranging from fasting to celery juice detox, brushing therapies, and many other interesting ideas. The people who care about us want nothing more than to help, but if she did everything they offered, she would be busy every minute of every day.

Gia knew her friends and family were trying to be helpful, but with the onslaught of external information, it had a "drinking from a firehose" effect. She questioned, "What matters? What doesn't? What's good for my cancer? How does anyone really know?" She thought dealing with her mental and emotional self was hard; the external information was mind-boggling.

BOB'S NEXT STEPS

A well-meaning family member even set an appointment with a local respected integrative oncologist for a second opinion. Bob was angry, but it was a favorite niece who arranged this, so he went, and it ended poorly.

Bob later told me that he went to the integrative oncologist for two reasons: one, for his favorite niece and two, on the off chance that integrative oncology had some secret he hadn't heard. Bob relayed that the physician said, "No cures unless your body does it, Bob, but we can offer improved quality of life, likely improved standard oncology therapy and possibly length of life." This is a very common and realistic response when a person has an advanced and aggressive cancer. Although there may be no "cure" for the cancer, there are often helpful therapies to improve the person's quality of life. None of this was what Bob wanted to hear. The physician later told me that in his thirty years of practice, Bob was the angriest patient he had ever seen.

THE PHYSICAL EXPERIENCE OF CANCER: A QUICK OVERVIEW

At this point, Bob had basically shut down, the external cancer process was going to "happen," and he was stepping out of the way. He was done. Nothing proactive was going to happen.

Gia realized from her inner work (and all the helpful ideas from friends and family) that there were many supportive ideas to consider. The trouble was that she had too many, and she became overwhelmed. She needed some clarity and a way to prioritize.

Although this book is intended to focus on the mental and emotional side of the cancer journey, there are things related to the physical aspects of cancer that are critical to your experience and outcomes. Aside from reading the book Dr. Stengler and I wrote, *Outside the Box Cancer Therapies*, I'll briefly outline important aspects of the physical cancer process while weaving in the mental and emotional aspects of your journey.

THE THREE PILLARS OF CANCER CARE

At roughly the two-decade mark of my practice, the National Institutes of Health research study was concluding. This gave me some time, and pause, to look at patterns I saw in patient survival, quality of life, and other factors associated with cancer. In looking back on people with cancer who survived versus people who did not, I saw a pattern appearing in those with similar types of cancer, especially in people who had a poor response to standard therapies due to cancer aggressiveness. As I studied the cases of these patients, I saw three basic pillars of health that emerged as precursors toward a tendency to survival or death. These became the Three Pillars upon which we based all other therapies. These pillars apply to standard of care cancer therapies as well as to all integrative, adjunctive, natural, or other therapies. I will describe each, but for memory sake, when I am teaching medical students and doctors, I use a three-word mnemonic: Food-Brain-Muscle.

These three factors (Food-Brain-Muscle) made the difference between survival and death in the worst cases. I now tell physicians and students, "You can do all the cool and high-tech medical interventions you want, but if they do not address these three areas, the other therapies will literally fall through the cracks and stop working."

1. FOOD

Food includes what we eat, the quantity and forms of food, the timing, and the cleanliness of the food (and drink).

2. BRAIN

Your mental and emotional world; what and who you let influence you; your level of mental toxicity or health; and your outlook and attitude. Simply put, the focus of this book.

3. MUSCLE

More muscle activity and less fat activity is associated with longer life, better survival, and improved quality of life in cancer patients (and most other people).

THE FOUR PARTS OF ANY CANCER JOURNEY

Similar to the Three Pillars of Food-Brain-Muscle, there are four distinct phases of the cancer journey. It is important to remember that these four phases are the same for standard oncology therapies as well as for integrative therapies. Understanding this helps in therapeutic decision making and is also empowering to you, the patient, as you make sense of the overwhelming process of having cancer. As a note, these are very brief descriptions. Much more detail (usually full chapters) is included in our book, *Outside the Box Cancer Therapies*.

1. PRIMARY PREVENTION

If you have cancer already, you are beyond this stage. Primary prevention is literally the initial and ongoing prevention of cancer. It is a part of the cancer journey as we all create potential cancers in our bodies daily but our immune systems (or related processes) remove them. The Three Pillars of Food-Brain-Muscle are critical in most primary prevention strategies.

2. DIAGNOSIS THROUGH ACTIVE TREATMENT

This is when the cancer is discovered (which often started months to years prior), and the initial therapies are offered and employed in your cancer care. This is often an intense, confusing, and very physically distressing time for patients.

3. RECOVERY FROM ACTIVE THERAPY

No matter the therapy (surgery, chemotherapy, radiation, etc.), the treatment often takes a toll on the body, which needs repair and recovery. This can be a time of mixed feelings as you may be hoping for a remission but at the same time may feel horrible. Physical fatigue and pain are common, as are depression, frustration, angst, and other emotional symptoms.

4. SECONDARY PREVENTION

Your mind and body have worked hard, the doctors have done their best, and now you may be in "remission" or been told you have "no evidence of disease." Awesome! This is certainly a time to celebrate, and you should. One caution after seeing things change (and in my experience, this is one of the biggest mistakes made), do not assume you are done with cancer. This is a time to work diligently to maintain your remission. If you simply say, "I'm done" and go back to the physical, mental, and emotional patterns prior to your diagnosis, in my experience, you commonly will not stay in remission.

YOUR NEXT STEPS

Empower yourself with knowledge.

Knowledge is power, and knowing what is likely next is empowering. I suggest reviewing the Three Pillars of cancer care and the section about the four parts of any cancer journey. You can use these ideas to look forward and locate your "true north" motivation in each area of your cancer journey. One example where knowledge is helpful involves understanding that a particular stage you are going through may be incredibly fatiguing, which can lead to a depressed mental state. Knowing that there is a physical reason for it allows you to get help for the physical part (something integrative oncology practitioners are excellent at doing) and perhaps have less worry over the way you feel.

Knowledge and information truly lead to personal empowerment. Empowerment leads to better all-around outcomes. You may indeed feel the steps outlined in this book provide you with some idea of a better path for you or your loved one's cancer journey.

But what if the one with cancer is my child? What can I do?

CHAPTER 8

I'M A PARENT OF A CHILD WHO HAS CANCER— WHAT DO I DO?

A CANCER DIAGNOSIS IS BAD, BUT HAVING YOUR CHILD DIAGNOSED WITH CANCER IS HELL

"You never know how strong you are until being strong is the only choice you have."

—CAYLA MILLS

You may not be dealing with a child who has cancer and this chapter may not appeal to you. That is completely fine. But as I work with families and children with cancer, it is a difficult situation and one that needs some special information.

Sadly, childhood cancer rates are on the rise. This chapter is for the children and their families to discuss the special circumstances they have.

(I will close out the stories of Bob and Gia in the next chapter.)

As a father, grandfather, and a physician who has walked with families of children who have had cancer, I think that the possibility of having a child diagnosed with cancer is one of the most difficult things to imagine. It's human nature to objectify such occurrences and think, "I'm glad it hasn't happened to me," but when childhood cancer touches your family, everything changes.

Childhood cancer has all the same variables as adult cancer: from treatable, curable, and hopeful to aggressive and lethal. In turn, children with cancer have all the modifying inner potential as adults.

In families of children who have cancer, everything discussed in the book applies, but it is multiplied from the patient to the parents, siblings, and other family members. It becomes a true community effect. All the complexities of family dynamics and differing worldviews can come crashing together. All the ideas and advice in the previous chapters still apply.

Below, I will relate some specific pediatric cancer ideas and strategies that I have seen help firsthand. First, I will relate my personal experience with cancer in children.

MY EXPERIENCE WITH PEDIATRIC CANCER

I have worked with children and their families through many pediatric cancers. I have rejoiced with families when their child achieved a remission. I have treated babies born with cancer and teenagers who developed sudden lethal cancers. I have sat with children and families in hospitals while the child passed away. And I have experienced everything in between.

I do not like cancer. I do not know anyone who does. I especially do not enjoy the process of cancer in a child and the effect it has on their family. However, it is a part of what I do because fewer physicians work with children than adults, and it is an area of great need. I will briefly relate two specific experiences in working with children with cancer.

As a doctor, when a patient dies, it is never pleasant, but it is something you adjust to as part of the job. When it is a child who dies, however, you never really adjust. Over two decades ago, I was working with a family and their child. The child was a twelve-year-old boy named Billy who had a brain tumor. In traditional cancer care, we did not have a great deal of success with these types of cancer, so I was working with Billy and the family on integrative cancer therapies to see if we could either improve his quality of life or extend his life. The therapies I included in Billy's care were "state of the art" at the time, and I would later be considered an innovator in these therapies. We worked hard with Billy and tried all our best therapies. Sadly, despite the best efforts from both standard and integrative cancer care, Billy lost his battle with this brain tumor and eventually died.

The death of Billy set me on a path to discover what we could do to improve cancer care. Even though there is no cure for cancer, both the standard and integrative worlds of cancer care evolve over time. What drives this innovation and evolution is the idea that "people who have cancer die, and we have to do better."

Fast forward twenty years. Another family with a child affected by a deadly cancer contacted me. When we met, they introduced me to their beautiful four-year-old daughter, Lilly. She was diagnosed at eleven weeks of age with a severe form of cancer. She had early treatment and had been in remission until now. She had fallen out of remission, and her only option was the same treatment that got her into remission the first time. The trouble was that certain blood markers were abnormal, and she could not receive the potentially lifesaving treatment until her blood markers normalized. The real problem was that there were no treatments in standard cancer care that could get her blood counts to normal. The family and our team were in a conundrum and needed to find a way to get her blood counts normalized so she could qualify for the other therapy.

Lilly was a delight to work with and to know. Her tiny blonde presence was the source of limitless joy, personality, and life. She lifted everyone around her and became an uplifting fixture at our clinic.

In the two decades since Billy's death, I had been involved in a great deal of innovative clinical cancer practice. That led to work in a federally funded cancer research project where I had the opportunity to try innovative cancer therapies as well as track those therapies to see if they work. When I met Lilly, I had been working in this program for a few years and had brought many of the innovations of the past decades to our integrative cancer practice.

We went to work and tried a therapy that failed. Then tried another that also failed. We tried more innovative therapies, and they failed. We tried combining some of the therapies, and that strategy failed as well. Lilly's blood counts were getting worse, and our therapies were not helping. There was a therapy that made complete sense "on paper" (from a scientific point of view), but we had tried it with only one person. It was helping that one person, but they were an adult and had a different kind of cancer. We were out of ideas and options, so I proposed this new therapy to the family.

When I proposed this new therapy idea, they said, "So you have tried this on one person so far?" "Yes," I replied, "and it has been safe and makes a lot of scientific sense." They continued saying, "And this is an adult who has a different cancer from Lilly?" I had to agree this seemed very "outside the box," but it was the only option I could see trying next. The look from them was "please tell us you are joking and that you have a better idea." I was not, and I did not.

The family and I decided to proceed. We knew there were no other options, and our only goal was to get her blood markers normal so she could have the other therapy. Without getting her blood markers back to normal, she would lose any chance of receiving the other therapy and really lose any chance for living very much longer.

We began the new therapy, and she responded very well. It was safe, well tolerated, and her blood markers were back to normal within three weeks. We kept the therapy going, and her blood markers remained normal. Thinking this may be a fluke, we stopped the therapy for a week, and her blood markers were abnormal again. We had two trials without the therapy, and both times her blood markers were not controlled. After that, we never stopped the experimental therapy again, because it worked. Her normal blood markers allowed her to start the standard therapy. To prepare her body, we also did some integrative treatment, another innovation of the years prior.

After this, the standard therapy worked, and Lilly went into remission. She responded well to the treatment, and we were ecstatic. We continued the original experimental therapy to keep her in remission and to keep her blood markers normal. The goal was to keep the latent cancer cells quiet and nonfunctional. Finally, the whole plan was working together, and she had some time that was relatively normal and healthy with her family.

Three years in remission had passed, and Lilly was living a relatively healthy and happy life. Then, as happens with severe genetically based cancers, the cancer figured out a way around the therapies and became active again. This time, the cancer came back forcefully. We quickly started to try innovative therapies to get her back into remission. We came close, and another standard therapy was tried. That standard therapy did not help, and her cancer progressed. Ultimately, as nothing was working, an experimental chemotherapy was tried. During this treatment she died, not from the cancer but due to side effects of the chemotherapy.

I was in her hospital room as she was passing away. Her family was around her, and even though it was a difficult time, it was also a touching and beautiful time for her transition. Her family asked if I would speak at her memorial service, which was an extreme honor. Lilly packed many decades of life and love into her eight years.

If the story ended there, for either Billy or Lilly, it would just be a sad story. The real benefit of their (and all the other patients') stories is what I learned from them. Their journeys made me more compassionate, more innovative, more aware, and a better doctor.

YOUR NEXT STEPS

In chapter 10, I am going to relate the real-world advice from two families who have lived the pediatric cancer journey. Their wisdom and ideas have come from living it. First, I will briefly relay some key points I have seen for parents and families of children with cancer.

Realize you have a "double portion" of the grief process.

You are processing your shock and grief as you engage in doing whatever you can for your child. Simultaneously, your child, regardless of age, is going through the process at an age-appropriate level. You are not only parenting while hurting, but you are also parenting a child with extreme health needs as well as deep mental and emotional needs. As one parent told me, "If you think parenting is difficult, try it with cancer thrown on top."

Be a light for your child to process all that is happening.

As with many things in parenting, you need to walk the line of caring for yourself and putting the needs of your child before yours. This is never easy. With cancer, you must elevate this in such a way that you are there for your child and can be a guide and light to them as they process it all in their own age-appropriate way. Although difficult, it can be done in a way that preserves your sanity and empowers your child. What I have seen work best is when the parent uses many of the strategies mentioned in the prior chapters and seeks some expert guidance regarding specific actions for their child. More on this in chapter 10 as well.

Understand that not all processing is verbal.

In younger children, we expect nonverbal (more emotional) processing. Of course, when they are not speaking yet, we see this as normal. But in my experience, it is the older verbal child who can surprise you with their nonverbal processing. At five or ten years of age, or even as a teenager, they will be processing in ways that overwhelm their conscious and verbal circuits. They often have mood swings, have anger and rage issues, withdraw, or act out in a variety of other ways. As I recommend for adults, professional help is critical for the child as well. There are mental health professionals who not only specialize in pediatrics but also cancer and chronic illness. They can be invaluable for support during this part of the journey.

Know that the process may be difficult, but it is still crucial.

Although I am making general statements, I have observed several responses to be consistent among children with cancer. Preverbal children are going to process it very simply and at a basic needs level. They often fear the unusual experiences (doctors, procedures, medicine, etc.) and do not like the pain. Early verbal children will usually process in "waves" at their specific level. They can be happily simplistic in their process and then come out with the most poignant and deep statements. These deeper thoughts are their less cluttered (than us adults) filter relating where in the process they are. Most parents are "there" for their children. Remember, as you are processing through your shock, grief, anger, or other emotions, your child needs as much of you as you can give.

In addition to the above ideas, I find there is no better advice than from those who have walked this road as parents of children with cancer. In chapter 10, with permission, I am including interviews with two families of pediatric cancer patients I have seen in my practice.

CHAPTER 9

NOW I HAVE SOME CLARITY, BUT I NEED RESOURCES AND TOOLS

"You can be a victim of cancer or a survivor of cancer. It's a mindset."

—DAVE PELZER

BOB AND GIA: BRINGING THEIR STORIES FULL CIRCLE

Since Bob and Gia are based on real people and you have been following their journeys in the chapters above, I think it is fitting to let you know how things progressed for them.

GIA'S CONCLUDING STEPS

Gia progressed through her mental and emotional process throughout her diagnosis and active cancer care. Her recovery from care was excellent, and she is now in secondary prevention maintaining her remission. At the time of this writing, she is over five years in remission. She continues to have her daily centering and gratitude practices and is always looking for more resources to continue to expand her empowerment journey. She knows that her job is to stay as healthy as possible: mentally, emotionally, and physically.

In addition to her gratitude practice, she has started an online resource for people with cancer to encourage and inform them. She finds this to be more rewarding than anything she has done, and her story gives her a great deal of credibility.

She works on the Three Pillars of Food-Brain-Muscle. Her life is precious, and she values every moment.

BOB'S CONCLUDING STEPS

Although some may have a hard time believing that Bob was a real person except for the name and a few details, he is 100 percent real. Bob went on and never changed his outlook or attitude. In fact, he became angrier over time.

He became very ill and progressed quickly. He was in pain, was taking a lot of pain medicine, and was obviously affected mentally by the heavy pain medicine doses.

Bob was in such pain, and such a state of misery, that he wanted to exercise what he thought was the last bit of control over his life. After months of suffering, he decided there was only one way out of his pain. One evening, alone in his home, he gave himself a carefully designed combination of medications. He no longer wanted to face his cancer diagnosis, and to him, ending his life was the only path he could see out of his pain and suffering. That evening, after taking his specially designed cocktail, Bob passed away.

As mentioned throughout this book, it is important to remember that this was Bob's life, and his alone. Although I feel sad for Bob and his family, I hold no judgment over him or his decisions. Ultimately, we answer to ourselves for our decisions and choices.

Would a change in his mental and emotional state have helped him? We cannot know for sure. That said, I do know other people with his type of cancer who did make drastic shifts and are still alive (beating the dismal 3–5 percent potential survival rate for his type of cancer).

SPECIFIC TOOLS

Tools can help address the most common places people get stuck, or when they have reversals during their cancer journey.

First, this chapter cannot address all the potential resources available. The goal of this section is to provide some of the most helpful tools to get started or to refine your own journey.

Second, I would like to point out something that you may have noticed as missing and wondered why. What you may have noticed missing is a discussion of a corollary to mental and emotional aspect of health often called spiritual. In my experience, many or most people have some spiritual leanings or background, and some do not. Some have spiritual changes when they confront their mortality as a result of a cancer diagnosis.

If you are a person who has, or is developing, a spiritual practice, it is yours and may be different from others in your friend and family group. The best thing I have seen is for you to incorporate your spiritual practice in the work you do for your mental and emotional processing. Please do not take the lack of depth on this massive subject as a lack of respect for the spiritual; in my experience, it is a profound factor in health and healing. Rather, please incorporate your spiritual work into the process outlined in this book and you will find synergy in many places.

I have listed some things to focus on in the Your Next Steps section. But first, I would like to respond to two questions I often hear.

WHAT IF I GET INTO REMISSION OR HAVE NO EVIDENCE OF DISEASE?

These are (aside from a miraculous cure) some of the best things that can happen in the cancer journey. When they do happen, the first thing is to give thanks for the outcome. Not everyone has the opportunity to achieve that status. The other thing is to remember that the steps you took to get there should be maintained to keep you there. Although cause for celebration, it should not be a reason to undo your diet, lifestyle, or mental and emotional work. Yes, celebrate! And then focus your energy on maintaining the new positive status.

WHAT IF THINGS AREN'T GOING WELL?

One question I hear commonly is, "If my cancer is that bad, why should I even try?" My first answer is that the decision of what work and how much work to do is completely up to you. Nobody can tell (or compel) you to do this work! My second answer is that if you are interested in any of the work suggested, you should do it regardless of the potential outcome of your cancer. I have seen countless cases where people were sent home to die, given weeks to months to live, and then have watched them live one, five, fifteen years. Sometimes even longer. Remember, a poor prognosis with cancer is based on statistics, not on you.

As mentioned, people who have cancer do pass away. Sometimes when all the "right" things are done and you have all your mental and emotional aspects the way you desire them, you may still be terminal. And no one knows for sure if a person will die prematurely from cancer, even in situations where it is certain. So what then?

Just like the different responses of Bob and Gia, I believe that you are in full control of your responses. I also believe you have the complete right to choose the way you decide to proceed. However, if things are not going well health-wise, you can decide to be as centered, happy, and emotionally fulfilled as you can be in the days that remain. I have seen people give up at this point and degenerate. I have also seen people live a new kind of joy and bliss in their final days. After doing their work, they seem to find a sense of peace knowing they did all they could and that every moment remaining would be precious.

Ultimately, it is completely up to you, but you can use the guidelines in this book to help you from the beginning to the end of the process.

YOUR NEXT STEPS

How does one go from processing the mental and emotional journey to maintaining and growing through the process?

The above chapters outline the how of getting through the initial process of self-assessment, getting help, staying on track, and taking a deeper look at the why. From there, as you approach the acceptance/empowerment stage, you now have more (but very rewarding) work ahead. Staying focused is key. The following ideas and the resource list provided will help keep you moving forward.

Find your "True North".

Finding your center or "true north" is critical to maintain your why and focus through the process. Life is hard, and life with cancer can be harder. You need to be clear as to why you want to go through the trouble of self-assessment and discovery. Why are you willing to grow personally while dealing with an often-overwhelming illness? All of this is difficult, especially at first, but your life can depend on you doing this work. (See the book by Dr. Samantha Brody, *Overcoming Overwhelm*. Information on this book can be found in the Resources section.)

Develop a gratitude practice.

A gratitude practice is just that—a practice of being grateful for every-thing we have. In my experience, gratitude helps people with cancer stay centered. Whether bad news or good news, gratitude helps people live every day enjoying what they do have. It can start by simply looking around you and giving thanks for anything you see that is a blessing. It may be a roof over your head, food, family, friends—all are a great start. This will reinforce your why and "true north" work.

Define success for yourself.

Through this process you'll want to identify what success means on your journey with cancer. Is it remission or no evidence of disease? Is it a cure? Is it living your best quality and quantity of life no matter what? This is woven into your why or "true north." You need to ask these questions and be honest when you find the answers.

Embrace and abandon outcomes.

In addition to defining what success means to you, a clear focus on things you can and sometimes cannot control is essential. I believe it is critical to maintain a good attitude, keep your sights and focus on healing, and live your best life. I also see people have worse outcomes when they get news that is not what they want or expected. For example, it is common for people to wait for the next marker (lab tests, imaging studies, examination, etc.) and put all their hope in the results. But then, if the news is not the best possible outcome, they become depressed and crestfallen and place their health in more jeopardy.

Yes, you want to visualize, plan for, and embrace the best of all outcomes. However, you also must know that whatever the intermediate outcome that is presented (better or worse lab tests, imaging, etc.), if you are still alive, you need your outlook to stay forward thinking and positive to keep progressing. The temporary negative news, poor experience, or outcome is a place along the way. It is not the end of the way.

Life continues as you go through the journey. We all have to accept that we are going to get good and bad news, and neither can be the reason we are up or down. If we do not accept that life happens, our life will be a never-ending roller coaster of emotion, and that does not correspond with the best outcomes or interests. Certainly, it is important to be realistic and understand that good or bad news is what it is, but it is not the beginning or the end of who you are or what is happening. As Dr. Frankl said, there is that moment between what happens (stimulus) and your response in which you do have a choice. It can feel good to choose to be angry, sad, or depressed. But you are the only one who can choose your response.

Although the storylines of Bob and Gia are complete (as far as this book is concerned), there are some resources and perspectives I believe will benefit you as you process your own journey. The chapters that follow are included to give you real patient and family feedback and also provide you with resources you may wish to use to deepen your understanding of areas mentioned in prior chapters.

CHAPTER 10

PATIENTS AND FAMILY MEMBERS TELL THEIR STORIES AND OFFER SOME INSIGHT

In this chapter, I am including four interviews with patients or family members. Two are adults and two are families of children with cancer. There is no replacement for the wisdom we can gain from people who have been there. I have kept the words as true to their own voice as possible. I will let their stories, advice, and love come through all on its own for you.

DAVID—LOVED ONE AND SUPPORT PERSON

At the center of my experience was the mental and emotional sphere. Mentally, I was overloaded with information, names, medicines, appointments, etc. Moreover, the constant oscillation between feeling how eagerly I wanted some moments to be done, while wishing others would last forever. The emotional side simply was overwhelming. I say that cautiously, because so many parts of our journey were emotionally overwhelming in the best way possible. The laughs, the tears, the feeling of togetherness, all the emotional experiences which I wouldn't trade for the world. Nothing else mattered. The only thing I put mental space against was my dad's care and well-being; the only thing I emotionally cared about was bringing all of his family together to create experiences while we could.

WHAT SURPRISED YOU MOST ABOUT OTHER PEOPLE'S REACTIONS?

Many people don't know what to say. Initially, I was very turned off that people would somewhat breeze over the topic. After all, it was my entire life at the time. I later learned that many people simply don't know what or how to say the right thing, or anything at all. I was also surprised by "knights"—those people who show up in fantastic ways.

WHAT ADVICE WOULD YOU GIVE FAMILY, FRIENDS, AND SUPPORTERS OF SOMEONE WITH CANCER?

Be genuine and understanding. Hopefully, you have never been through anything as scary as what that person is experiencing— to pretend that you have is unfair. Most importantly, however you related to that person before their diagnosis, relate to them in the same way after; just do so with a renewed sense of the value that person brings to your life.

I was lucky: the patient was my best friend and dad. During my experience with him, I made every effort to experience him as father and friend, not as someone in need of my care.

WERE THERE ANY RESOURCES YOU FOUND HELPFUL?

There were three resources I found helpful. My family and friends, Dr. Josh Trutt, and my own yoga/meditation practice.

IS THERE ANY OTHER ADVICE YOU FOUND TO BE HELPFUL IN YOUR PROCESS?

My cousin Mikey who had lost both his parents to cancer just a few years prior, told me something I will never forget: "Spend every possible moment with your dad." It was the best advice. I'm not sure I ever would have been able to find peace with his passing if I hadn't been present for every possible moment. Lastly, if the person you love is not on the course to recovery, look at them and remember who they are, what makes them so unique, so special and so loved by you. Don't look at them for what the disease has done to their body. There will be a moment, when you are looking at them for who they are, and they will look back and you will never forget it. I promise.

WHITNEY—A YOUNG WOMAN WITH A CANCER SO RARE THAT THERE ARE NO STATISTICS ABOUT HER CANCER OR OTHER COMMON "TOOLS" IN STANDARD ONCOLOGY TO RELY ON FOR HER PRIMARY TREATMENT

Prior to surgery, I needed a lot of alone time. I wanted to hide my pain from my family and act strong to ease their pain. I also needed to do my own thing and prepare for potentially my final days. I had two weeks between diagnosis and surgery, as that two-pound sucker (the tumor) had to come out *fast*. I chose my routine 2.6 mile run around my favorite lake, and I drove to every single one of my favorite beaches in Bellingham and screamed and bawled with the wind and waves. I let nature embrace my confusion and terror. My best friend did a photo shoot of me in a fabulous ball gown I bought and returned to Macy's. I checked off a major bucket list item and summited Mount Baker. I focused on myself. I fled to the hills and enjoyed the [heck] out of those two weeks.

For me, diagnosis, surgery, and recovery were the easy part. Regretfully, after surgery, the impact of chemotherapy and long-term treatment decision making really play games with your brain. I felt like a superstar coming out of surgery. I had survived the insurmountable and had no cancer. Everything—literally, everything—in surgery had gone exponentially better than possible. But instead of receiving support, care, empathy, understanding, and kindness from others, there was an overwhelming amount of destructive criticism and intense analysis around my "precancer" life and what could have possibly caused this disease in a young adult. People wanted to pick through my every move to decipher what had led to this event, when in fact, it was quite literally out of my control. Growing up from the age of eight with a parent with cancer, our family had gone above and beyond to adopt every healthy habit out there. I was raw vegan for two years prior to diagnosis, I made vision boards, I exercised every day, I had gone to an amazing counselor for ten years, I went to eating disorder support groups to address my issues with food, I saw countless nutritionists and fantastic naturopaths, and I always maintained a healthy weight, invested in self-care, and prioritized emotional, physical, and mental health to the best of my ability.

ARE YOU THE PATIENT OR A LOVED ONE/SUPPORT PERSON?

Both! My father was diagnosed with stage 3 prostate cancer when I was eight years old, about twenty years ago. From the moment I was diagnosed, there were tears, but there was also action. As a family unit, we knew exactly what to do. Proceed forward.

WHAT SURPRISED YOU MOST ABOUT YOUR MENTAL AND EMOTIONAL WORLD SHIFT AFTER YOU WERE DIAGNOSED?

What surprised me the most about my cancer diagnosis was not the initial surgery and treatment but the long-term haul. One of my doctors compared chemotherapy and return to health as a "marathon." Nothing has ever rung so true physically but especially mentally. Surgery was easy. The University of Washington (UW) was fantastic. However, no one prepares you for the long-term emotional haul. As a stage 3 patient on three-plus years of daily, oral, experimental chemotherapy, this slowly began to erode my concrete foundation. I ravaged my way through the initial first year post-op, and began chemo with incredible, hidden, tortured pain. From the moment I placed the pills on my tongue, I could feel my previously joyful brain slowly dull. This was a struggle others could empathize with but not understand. My vocal cords had turned a different, unrecognizable octave from tumor testosterone exposure, and now my brain, too, began to color life in a foreign haze. I no longer recognized my own brain, processing, or thinking.

WHAT SURPRISED YOU MOST ABOUT OTHER PEOPLE'S REACTIONS?

It frustrated me to no end when people would start crying and looking to support from me regarding my own diagnosis. While I understand they were grieving for me, and these emotions came from a place of love, next time, please get a room. I could barely navigate my own feelings, and you wanted me to help you handle yours as well? Did you expect me to support your grief as well as my own confrontation of mortality? These types of people are annoying. Ignore and avoid them as much as possible. You do not need their pity. You are powerful beyond your capacity and knowing.

It's such an insult when another person looks at my life with pity or sadness. Yes, I'm on some radically annoying drugs, but I made it out of an insane surgery with an intact liver, kidney, GI tract, lungs, and heart with no signs of metastatic disease! Yes, my prognosis is 15 percent, but I'm alive! There is so much to be grateful for. How dare you diminish my joy with your side glances of pity!

WHAT ADVICE WOULD YOU GIVE FAMILY, FRIENDS, AND SUPPORTERS OF PEOPLE WITH CANCER?

Embrace every moment. Don't cry on the patient or person with cancer. They don't need that guilt.

Get used to the sound of barfing and lots of talk of digestive issues.

WHAT ADVICE WOULD YOU GIVE SOMEONE IN YOUR OWN SHOES WHO IS JUST ENTERING THE WORLD OF A CANCER JOURNEY?

When you are hit with a cancer diagnosis, everyone and their distant relative seems to gain an MD/ND/PhD in cancer treatment or cell biology and will overload you with any and every article and information possible. Slow your roll, people. I think the best thing I found was to go with my own instinct. And surround yourself with people who support you in that endeavor. My cousin, in particular, 110 percent supported me in pursuing whatever form of cancer treatment I wanted and felt best. This was the most helpful.

Many people will make you feel guilty unintentionally. This cancer was not your fault. Cancer does not pick and choose. Don't judge yourself. Don't compare yourself to other people's cancer difficulties. So many times, I would look on social media and get incredibly depressed from other people's life trajectories. Your path is just as gorgeous, however long and however many scars.

PEDIATRIC CANCER

The following are shared by two families who have experienced life with a child with cancer. It is with extreme gratitude that I received their feedback, and they both want their stories to continue to help other families who have children dealing with cancer.

THE STERNAGLES—PARENTS OF RYDER, A BOY WHO HAS AN INCREASINGLY MORE COMMON CANCER FOUND IN CHILDREN

The mental and emotional aspect has played a huge role on multiple fronts. Likely the biggest has been perseverance and mental toughness. We've sought to do what we think and feel to be *the right thing* at every step of the journey, yet that choice has always led to the path of most resistance. It's taken a lot of willpower and resolve to stick to each and every one of those decisions, but we're so glad we have, as they've all paid off beyond what we could have imagined. Moving states to be with a more cooperative and supportive medical team, stopping conventional treatment halfway through the standard of care as parents of a pediatric cancer patient, deciding to go deeper and deeper into debt to obtain all the out-of-pocket complementary treatments and other factors related to his wellness we could, building a nontoxic house in the middle of the woods to be in complete control of his environment, and so on, have all been what most would consider to be decisions they would not have been able to bring themselves to make. And aside from added work, each of them has come with a whole lot of scrutiny from friends, family, and everyone who follows our story. However, we've watched so many others accept the default conditions presented to them, which is always following what seems to be the path of least resistance up front, but what it seems to lead to is a downward spiral that's much harder to climb back out of in the long run.

It's also important to note that closely related to this perseverance has been some form of visualization, even if we haven't necessarily called it that along the way. We've spent so much time talking about everything we've wanted to accomplish, obtain, follow through with, etc., before it ever happened, and so far, it all has.

Lastly, as a caregiver and parent, we've noticed a direct correlation with our mental state and the level of care Ryder receives. We joke that early on, we looked more like the cancer patients than he did, as we were pouring all of ourselves into him, and any modicum of attention paid to our own well-being seemed selfish. However, if we could go back and change anything, it would likely be our attitude. The better care we take of ourselves, combined with the most positive outlook we're able to maintain, always results in Ryder getting all of his supplements, fitting all of his therapies in, and all around looking, feeling, and acting the best himself. The only time his care slips is when we slip out of the best mental and physical state.

WHAT SURPRISED YOU MOST ABOUT YOUR MENTAL AND EMOTIONAL WORLD SHIFT AFTER RYDER WAS DIAGNOSED?

It's not an uncommon answer, but our priorities radically shifted. We were both very into what was going on in the world, how and why things are the way they are, and so on. Probably a year after diagnosis, I figured I'd see what was going on in the world and realized the app I used to check the news was so far out of date it had stopped working. Instead of updating it, I took it as a sign and probably went another whole year without really caring what was happening.

WHAT SURPRISED YOU MOST ABOUT OTHER PEOPLE'S REACTIONS?

What surprised us most about others' reactions to our son's

diagnosis was the near avoidance from so many that we had considered to be varying levels of close friends or acquaintances in our lives, combined with the overwhelming generosity and care from so many we'd never met.

In taking the road less traveled, so to speak, a lot of folks saw that as taking our son's life into our own hands, which was perceived to be a negative thing that they didn't want to be involved with. Others came forward later and said that with small children of their own, it hit too close to home. Others just didn't know how to handle it and chose to do nothing at all.

At the same time, though, we were really putting ourselves out there in a big way on social media, to raise as much money as we could to continue to support Ryder at the same levels, and to spread what we were learning about healing holistically to as many other parents and patients as we could. We were blown away, almost daily, at how many otherwise complete strangers resonated with what we were doing and flooded us with all forms of support, from monetary to emotional to services, to things we didn't even know we needed until someone thought to help us with them.

WHAT ADVICE WOULD YOU GIVE FAMILY, FRIENDS, AND SUPPORTERS OF PEOPLE WITH CANCER?

Let them know you care and are thinking about them. Not just once but repeatedly. Even if you don't hear back from them.

They're going through a whole lot and remembering to respond can very easily fall through the cracks, but knowing that they're not alone, and that others care about what happens to them, can mean more than you'll ever realize.

Also, whenever possible, don't tell them what you're going to do for them. Do it, and then tell them what you did. It's really easy to say you're going to do something for someone, much harder to follow through. It can be really disheartening to get told something is going to be done for you, only to shortly thereafter wonder if it's ever really going to happen. On the other hand, being told about something that was just done for you is one of the best feelings in the world. It doesn't have to be big things either (although probably the most impactful thing you could do would be to organize a fundraiser outside of whatever they're currently doing). Mow their lawn, clean their house, watch their kids, ask for their grocery list the day you know you'll be at the grocery store—there are lots of little things you can do that take a huge burden off of them and allow them to focus on healing.

WERE THERE ANY RESOURCES YOU FOUND HELPFUL?

Naturopathic Oncology by Neil McKinney and *The Definitive Guide to Cancer* by Lise Alschuler are particularly useful in considering various supplements and complementary treatments in conjunction with conventional treatment. *Outside the Box Cancer Therapies* by Paul Anderson is the best book to get a complete protocol to start the journey.

When you start diving into the world of holistic/integrative treatment, there's way more out there to choose from than you could ever implement at one time or even over a long period of time. Let intuition be your ultimate guide. At some level, you do know exactly what you (or even your kid) need(s); the more you can tap into that and trust it, the better your decision-making process will become.

No one's coming to save you. You are the only person that can save yourself or your child. People might care a whole lot about you, but no one cares about your survival more than you do, and no one is in a better position to implement all the measures that can help you than you are. But this isn't about going it alone. Ask for as much help as you possibly can, for everything you possibly can, from as many people as you possibly can.

THE HULTBERGS—PARENTS OF LILLY, A CHILD WHO HAD A VERY AGGRESSIVE TYPE OF CHILDHOOD LEUKEMIA

(I wrote about her in the chapter on children.)

WHAT PLACE HAS THE MENTAL AND EMOTIONAL SPHERE PLAYED IN YOUR CANCER JOURNEY?

Fear: I don't look at a common cold or flu the same way. My mind immediately jumps to the worst possible situation. I can tell you that I've had my boys' blood drawn to check for low platelets, etc., because they've had a bruise that they or I couldn't figure out how they got. Even with myself I've asked for tests to be done to check things out because I've let the fear of cancer take over. In my mind, I feel if you let your shoulders down, then cancer will strike again. After all, it has no boundaries. Cancer doesn't care who you are or how old you are—it just seeks and destroys.

WHAT SURPRISED YOU MOST ABOUT YOUR MENTAL AND EMOTIONAL WORLD SHIFT AFTER LILLY WAS DIAGNOSED?

Lots of things. For starters, my ability to keep going. On what, I have no idea. I look back now and think, "Was that life even real?" I was consumed by blood counts. I would study those lab reports over and over. One, hoping they would change if I looked at them hard enough and two, trying to come up with an explanation of why they were how they were. I realized soon our lives were forever changed. I felt the need to keep my whole family in a "clean bubble" for fear someone would get sick and Lilly's immune system wouldn't be able to fight it off.

Another thing that surprised me is how many people cared. We had so many people, some we knew really well, others were just acquaintances, and some were complete strangers, that reached out to help us. It's a humbling experience. I can say I wish we didn't have to go through what we did to witness such "giving," but I know we wouldn't have been able to get through it if we didn't have so many people reaching out to help. I can also tell you that my faith shifted. I think this is the point where you think I'm going to say my faith grew stronger, that I could feel God's presence with us at all times. That was not the case. I can say there were times that I felt very alone. I questioned God and why He chose Lilly to go through something so horrific. I can look back now and see God's hand and His direction for not just Lilly but our whole family. I guess you could say I'm still a work in progress on my faith. I'll never understand why Lilly had to have cancer for almost all of her life and then ultimately die. It's something I'm sure I'll understand one day when I'm reunited with Lilly in heaven.

WHAT ADVICE WOULD YOU GIVE FAMILY, FRIENDS, AND SUPPORTERS OF PEOPLE WITH CANCER?

First, never, ever say, "I know what you're going through." Everyone's journey is different. Everyone deals with their experience differently. I also think it's important to keep in contact with them. The outside "normal" world is no longer existing. It's nice to hear things about where you are living, what's going on. I would, however, advise you not to complain about your daily life and how hard it is. I can remember talking to a friend while in the hospital with Lilly and she was complaining how tired she was from taking kids to school and helping with homework, doing laundry, and cooking dinner. She was upset because she had little time for herself. I remember thinking, "I would give anything to live that life."

WHAT ADVICE WOULD YOU GIVE SOMEONE IN YOUR OWN SHOES WHO IS JUST ENTERING THE WORLD OF A CANCER JOURNEY?

Take a breath. Be positive. Have a mindset of cancer not winning. Do whatever it takes. Go beyond your comfort zone to seek treatment. Pray. The best advice I ever got, which I still use today: Hang in there. Be Bold. Be confident. It's OK to ask questions. It's OK to have people help you. It's OK to feel angry and sad and cry. I think it's even good to have those feelings. Use that anger and direct it to a positive energy. When you're sad, give yourself a day to be sad! Wake up the next day ready to fight. Don't jump down the sad rabbit hole; you'll never get out. Laugh! Laugh as much as you can. Above all, never, ever, ever give up!

Every effort was taken to limit editing of these brave contributions. Edits were made for style and flow, but the rest are their stories, as told. There could be many comments, clarifications, or explanations added, but after reading these gifts of others' human experiences with the cancer journey, I made the decision to let every word, thought, feeling, and emotion stand as is for all of you to take in.

CHAPTER 11

RESOURCES

This chapter provides easy access to techniques, references, and resources to reinforce and enhance your implementation of the work done throughout this book. This book could have been ten times longer, but so many great resources already exist that I have chosen to point you to them here.

The first points are tips for dealing with common issues that come up in this journey. Then there are some resources and links to look at if you want to dive deeper into the material. Finally, a brief list of books I have used or patients have highly recommended.

DEALING WITH FAMILY AND FRIENDS
"I" STATEMENTS

Thomas Gordon is credited for developing the "I" statement in the 1960s as a style of communication that focuses on the feelings of the speaker rather than the characteristics the speaker attributes to the listener. Example: A person might say to their partner, "I feel abandoned and worried when you consistently come home late without calling," instead of demanding, "Why are you never home on time?" It can help neutralize the request by focusing on your needs and not the behavior of others.

This is more critical with some people in our lives than others but can open and deescalate communication with anyone. You have enough going on in your life that any advantage you can use to decrease stress in communication is important.

REINFORCING POSITIVE BEHAVIOR

When trying to shift the focus of behavior, the use of "I" statements are powerful. The use of reinforcement phrases with our family and friends are also powerful. This is essentially focusing on what we want to see in the relationship and, even if something small, finding things the other person is doing well and pointing them out. This is often the opposite of what many of us learn, which is pointing out the negative we do not desire. A reinforcing statement such as, "I love it when you ___" or "It makes my day when you support me by ___" can be incredibly powerful at showing others what helps us most.

If you were not raised using "I" statements or reinforcement, it can feel odd and forced at first. The benefit is that the communication around what you need is relayed in a neutral, nonjudgmental, and positive manner. This is normally a win for any relationship.

HOW DO I PROTECT MY INNER SELF FROM POISONOUS THOUGHTS AND INFLUENCES?

We have spoken about toxic people, relationships, and situations. Most people realize that toxicity in human interactions can be more damaging to health than a toxic chemical. Below, I have provided links to two brief essays regarding toxic interactions and strategies to manage these interactions. Every human has some level of toxic humanity around them, but being able to recognize and deal with it increases your empowerment and control over your health.

- https://www.scarymommy.com/dealing-with-toxic-people/
- https://www.psychologytoday.com/us/blog/in-flux/201608/8-things-the-most-toxic-people-in-your-life-have-in-common

A SMALL SELECTION OF RESOURCES FOR PEDIATRIC CANCER AND FAMILIES

The website the Sternagle family (featured in the patient stories section of this book) has developed to assist families who have children with cancer:

- https://thesternmethod.com/

How to tell children:

- https://www.cancer.org/treatment/children-and-cancer/
  when-a-family-member-has-cancer/dealing-with-
  diagnosis/how-to-tell-children.html
- https://blog.dana-farber.org/insight/2013/03/five-ways-to-
  support-families-dealing-with-childhood-cancer/
- https://www.huffpost.com/entry/15-things-parents-of-
  kids-with-cancer-want-you-to-know_n_57d728ede4b-
  09d7a687f503f
- https://www.cancer.org/latest-news/caring-for-children-
  with-cancer.html

BOOKS TO CONSIDER

I want you to find books and resources you resonate with and feed your process. These are some I am familiar with that reinforce the ideas in the chapters above. This list could be much longer, and my omission of an excellent book is not a judgment. The list of books below are ones that I and my patients have had the most experience with and benefit from.

Note that these are listed in alphabetical order by title.

- *The Biology of Belief 10th Anniversary Edition: Unleashing the Power of Consciousness, Matter & Miracles*, by Dr. Bruce H. Lipton

- *Breast Cancer: Thriving through Treatment to Recovery*, by Dr. Lisa A. Price
- *But It's Your Family…Cutting Ties with Toxic Family Members and Loving Yourself in the Aftermath*, by Dr. Sherrie Campbell
- *Cooking through Cancer Treatment to Recovery: Easy, Flavorful Recipes to Prevent and Decrease Side Effects at Every Stage of Conventional Therapy*, by Dr. Lisa Price and Susan Gins
- *The Honeymoon Effect: The Science of Creating Heaven on Earth*, by Dr. Bruce H. Lipton
- *It's OK that You're Not OK: Meeting Grief and Loss in a Culture that Doesn't Understand*, by Megan Devine
- *The Metabolic Approach to Cancer: Integrating Deep Nutrition, the Ketogenic Diet and Non-Toxic Bio-Individualized Therapies*, by Dr. Nasha Winters and Jess Higgins Kelley
- *Mindfulness-Based Cancer Recovery: A Step-by-Step MBSR Approach to Help You Cope with Treatment and Reclaim Your Life*, by Linda E. Carlson, PhD, and Michael Speca, PsyD, foreword by Zindel Segal, PhD
- *Naturopathic Oncology: An Encyclopedic Guide for Patients and Physicians*, by Dr. Neil McKinney
- *The Next Place*, by Warren Hanson (a book for children dealing with grief)
- *On Grief and Grieving: Finding the Meaning of Grief through the Five Stages of Loss*, by Elisabeth Kübler-Ross and David Kessler
- *Outside the Box Cancer Therapies*, by Drs. Mark Stengler and Paul Anderson

- *Overcoming Overwhelm: Dismantle Your Stress from the Inside Out*, by Dr. Samantha Brody
- *Prostate Cancer: Thriving through Treatment to Recovery*, by Dr. Lisa A. Price
- *Radical Remission*, by Kelly A. Turner
- *Self Care Isn't Selfish: Your Roadmap for Taking Responsibility for Your Own Happiness*, by Susie Ascott
- *Spontaneous Evolution: Our Positive Future and a Way to Get There from Here*, by Dr. Bruce H. Lipton
- *Textbook of Naturopathic Oncology*, by Dr. Gurdev Parmar
- *Thrive Don't Only Survive: Dr. Geo's Guide to Living Your Best Life before and after Prostate Cancer*, by Dr. Geo Espinoza

PROFESSIONAL ORGANIZATIONS

- Behavioral Resources for Oncology: https://www.bhthechange.org/resources/mental-health-impacts-of-a-cancer-diagnosis/
- Oncology Association of Naturopathic Physicians: https://oncanp.org/
- Society for Integrative Oncology: https://integrativeonc.org/
- Stages of Grief website: https://grief.com/the-five-stages-of-grief/

CONCLUSION

You CAN do this!

As difficult as it seems, you have the knowledge and power to take control of your mental and emotional state and use it to your advantage. It DOES make a difference.

There is no way to make this easy, but anyone can do this. And this work will dramatically change the way you feel and interact through your process with cancer.

I used the stories of Bob and Gia to illustrate the countless types of patients I have seen over the years and just how their internal work helped or hindered their progress. Yes, ultimately it is your choice as to how you do this, but this book is designed to help you find a better, healthier way based on what I have seen in practice. As I've said throughout this book, this isn't a theoretical or academic book. It's real. It's from my daily work with patients and families dealing with cancer.

Throughout the book I have talked about the roller coaster of feelings and emotions we all experience. Although everyone processes their own way (which is healthy and normal), there is a process that happens to everyone over time. The goal in looking at this was twofold: it is normal to process your own way and in as many cycles as needed, and understanding the process allows you to keep moving and find higher states of empowerment.

Together, we looked at how to deal with those around us—family and friends and how they are on their own internal journey. Too often, I have seen people moving through empowerment themselves but surrounded by confused or unhelpful family and friends. I made sure to write about how to deal with toxic people and how to set healthy boundaries with those who really want to help you.

The chapter about children with cancer was written from a great deal of personal experience. The statistics show childhood cancer is on the rise and most people will know or will be a family member of a child with cancer at some point in their lives. The interviews in chapter 10 with parents of children with cancer are invaluable.

Throughout this book, but specifically in the resources section, I have included tools and resources as a place to start if you want or need more information on a topic. The goal of this book is for you to have a base to work from and then discover areas you want to quickly explore further. And remember, this work is a process—so, you can read the book again and find new areas to focus on as you grow.

You CAN do this!

As difficult as it seems, you have the knowledge and power to take control of your mental and emotional state and turn it to your advantage. Is it easy? No. Is it important? Yes.

So what do I do now?

Whether you've read the entire book through, skipped through it, or read the conclusion first, I recommend you do the following:

1. Do a quick overview of the chapters/topics and write down the ones that speak the most to you where you are today.
2. Take each of those and ask: Is the chapter enough for me to get started? Do I need a deeper resource? What are the first things I need to do to explore that more and grow there?
3. Settle into that work, and as it progresses, you'll find new ideas and challenges open up for you. As they do, know that is normal and go back to step 1 above.

It's a process, and the goal is to improve your quality of life, happiness, health, and relationships regardless of a "diagnosis." So, "empowerment" is whatever you personally need to make this journey. You won't regret it!

And remember, you CAN do this.

With the greatest care, love, and empowerment for you and your process.

DR. PAUL ANDERSON

ACKNOWLEDGMENTS

For their wonderful editing and support: Dr. John Nowicki and Davindia Steele.

And for the patients and families who allowed me to interview them so their stories could be heard.

ABOUT THE AUTHOR

DR. PAUL S. ANDERSON is a nationally recognized educator and clinician with more than three decades of experience with cancer and complex chronic illness. As head of the interventional arm of a human trial funded by the US National Institutes of Health, Dr. Anderson oversaw research into integrative therapies for cancer patients.

Dr. Anderson was the founder of a number of clinics specializing in the care of people with cancer and chronic illness and is now focusing his efforts training other physicians and writing. He is the coauthor of *Outside the Box Cancer Therapies*, with Dr. Mark Stengler, and the anthology *Success Breakthroughs*, with Jack Canfield.

WHERE CAN I FIND DR. ANDERSON ONLINE?

Facebook: Dr. A Online
Instagram: DrAonline
Twitter: @DrPaulAnderson1
Website: DrAnow.com/DrAbooks.com

Printed in Great Britain
by Amazon

46599557R00081